Neal's Yard Natural Remedies

Susan Curtis, Romy Fraser
and Irene Kohler

ARKANA

ARKANA

Published by the Penguin Group
Penguin Books Ltd, 27 Wrights Lane, London W8 5TZ, England
Penguin Books USA Inc., 375 Hudson Street, New York, New York 10014, USA
Penguin Books Australia Ltd, Ringwood, Victoria, Australia
Penguin Books Canada Ltd, 10 Alcorn Avenue, Toronto, Ontario, Canada M4V 3B2
Penguin Books (NZ) Ltd, 182–190 Wairau Road, Auckland 10, New Zealand

Penguin Books Ltd, Registered Offices: Harmondsworth, Middlesex, England

First published in Great Britain by Arkana 1988
10 9 8 7 6 5 4

Printed in England by Clays Ltd, St Ives plc
Filmset in 11/12pt Ehrhardt Linotron

ARKANA

NEAL'S YARD
NATURAL REMEDIES

This book is written jointly by the owner of the Neal's Yard Remedies shops, Romy Fraser, and two of her colleagues, Susan Curtis and Irene Kohler, all of whom have several years' experience in working with natural remedies. Susan Curtis practises homoeopathy professionally, and all three authors have studied aromatherapy. Neal's Yard Remedies has made a huge impact since the shop first opened in Covent Garden, London. It is one of the pioneers of natural beauty products and natural health care. There are now several franchises throughout England, and the products are available in the United States and Australia.

Gini Wade

Grateful thanks for their valuable contributions are offered to: Ruby Cook, Dr Brian Kennedy and Annie McIntyre.

Contents

Introduction

We have worked together for several years from behind the counter at Neal's Yard Apothecary, unable to offer remedies that we feel would be appropriate for the complaints that people bring to us. There are two main reasons for this. The first is that we would be breaking the law; most of the remedies do not have a product licence and we are not allowed to recommend their usage. These remedies have stood the test of time, they have been used with great benefit for many years; but not all 'natural' remedies are safe to use, especially over prolonged periods of time and with a high dosage.

Second, we are only too aware that any single complaint may be a symptom of a whole imbalance in the body. It is not just the symptom that must be dealt with but the whole person, and the whole picture that can be built up can only be dealt with during a considered consultation with an experienced practitioner. It would therefore be irresponsible and impossible in the situation behind the counter to give a diagnosis and offer the appropriate remedy when we are busy serving customers, answering the telephone, and running our shops.

What we hope to achieve by writing this book is to give some ideas of safe and helpful remedies for common illness and first-aid. Much of our ill-health is a result of the way we live, combined with inherited factors. By writing this book we would like to enable our customers to increase their ability to make the choice of remedy for themselves. We have approached this in the form of a simple alphabetical repertory; but always, any chosen remedy should be cross-referenced by consulting the appropriate specialist books that we recommend in the Bibliography, to get a more complete picture of the remedy itself and its appropriateness for the complaint.

The whole question of ill-health and well-being is interesting. Why should we get ill? Whose responsibility is it? And what can we learn from it? Maybe if we had been more in touch with our bodies and noticed the odd warnings that we received, we would have avoided the greater discomfort that we often find ourselves in. We may enjoy a few drinks, cigarettes, running a home, and/or a demanding job, yet we continue to expect ourselves to remain fit, stress-free, and happy.

Encouraging our bodies towards an improved balance in health may involve changing our lifestyles. Do we want to do this? How much is it worth perpetuating a lifestyle that disturbs our well-being? Pollution, fast foods with additives, and the stress accumulated by the current values of society are continually pulling against a state of good health.

The process of becoming healthy offers the opportunity for growth and change. At times this process can be hindered or blocked by illness. In this book we can only offer solutions to some acute problems that are often the outcome of a temporary imbalance. When attitudes become fixed, then chronic complaints become established, and for these we will always recommend professional advice.

Something common to us all is the desire or drive to improve our lives, so here in this book our intention is to offer you the opportunity to take greater responsibility for your own discomfort or ill-health in a way that is safe and effective, but without the side-effects encountered when using synthetic drugs.

HERBS

Plants are an integral part of the cycle of life on this planet. Human beings entirely depend on plant life to sustain us: not only are plants the source of all our food, but they create the air we breathe and are the original source of all our medicines.

As life has become more complicated so too have the medicines we use. Modern society has largely replaced the use of healing plants — herbs — by sophisticated drugs. Currently, vast financial resources are being invested in the exploration and analysis of medicinal substances, often derivatives and synthetics based on plant constituents. However, in recent times, there is also a trend towards re-evaluating 'natural' medicine, and herbs are again being sought out for their intrinsic therapeutic properties.

The use of herbal medicine has been passed down through the centuries by those practised in the art of healing. These traditional remedies are coming to be sought after again as effective, safe and proven alternatives to our synthetic medicines. Herbs can be used to support the natural healing processes in the body; not just directly attacking the disease, which is the approach generally offered by modern drugs.

For minor ailments the herbs that we suggest may be tried, but for real benefit in more serious cases a qualified herbalist should be consulted, who can assess each case individually and adjust dosage as required.

GATHERING HERBS

The majority of herbs we have recommended in this book can be found growing wild. Care must be taken that they are collected some distance from roads and any other sources of pollution. Herbs can of course be cultivated (unless you live in a city), and collected and used when needed.

To dry herbs gather them just before they have fully developed, in dry weather, as soon as the dew has gone in the morning. Remove any dead or damaged parts of the plants and then spread the herbs out to dry in a dry, well-ventilated atmosphere.

STORAGE

Storage of your own herbs, or the ones that you purchase, should be away from light and in airtight jars. The effectiveness of herbalism depends greatly on the quality of the herbs used: they should look and smell fresh and bright.

PREPARING HERBS

Infusions

An infusion is made like tea, it is the suitable method for herbal mixtures of flowers, leaves and green stems. Place the herb or herbs in a pot, pour on boiling water, cover and leave to stand for ten minutes before straining.

The quantity of herb to use will vary according to the quality of the herb and the strength of the infusion required. A general guide is to use one tablespoon of herbs to a pint of boiling water, or one heaped teaspoon of herbs to a cupful of boiling water. When using fresh herbs double the quantity of herb to be used.

Herbal preparations can be taken hot or cold. Hot infusions will tend to encourage sweating, cold ones tend to be more diuretic. Therefore, use hot infusions to treat colds, 'flu, fevers etc., these may be sweetened with honey for taste. If in doubt, it is usually considered best to take medicinal teas hot.

Decoctions

For the harder, woodier roots and barks of plants it is necessary to make a decoction. Place the herb or herbs in a saucepan, pour on some water, bring to the boil and then simmer for ten to fifteen minutes before straining. Do not use an aluminium pan but a glass, ceramic or unchipped enamel one. This method is also suitable for berries and the harder seeds.

Use the same quantities as recommended for infusions although you may need to add a little more water to allow for evaporation.

Tinctures

Alcohol-based preparations are called tinctures. Tinctures tend to be stronger, volume for volume, than infusions or decoctions. Dosage should be from five to fifteen drops of tincture taken in a wine glass of water.

Compresses and Poultices

To make a compress, use a clean cloth and soak it in a hot infusion or decoction. Place this as warm as possible upon the affected area and either change it when it cools down or cover the cloth with a sheet of plastic and place a hot water bottle on this. The heat will enhance the activity of the herb.

To make a poultice use either fresh or dried herbs. With the fresh plant you apply the bruised leaves or root material either directly on the skin or place it between thin gauze. With the dried herb, first make a paste by adding hot water, then apply in the same way as a compress.

CAUTION

Herbalism is one of the oldest known ways of healing. The herbs we have suggested in this book have been used for centuries: they have passed the test of time, and are effective and often powerful. Although herbalism is a natural form of healing, this must not be confused with being entirely harmless. Herbs have a strong therapeutic value and they must be used with respect and common sense.

It is best to be cautious, and any problem that is severe or persists with the use of these herbs, should be taken to a qualified practitioner. It is unwise to continue using herbs over a prolonged period of time or to exceed a safe dose.

It is always advisable to cross-reference any herb that you intend to use with a herbal reference book (see the Bibliography).

HOMOEOPATHY

The word homoeopathy comes from the Greek, it means 'similar suffering'. It is based on the law of similars: that 'like cures like'. A homoeopathic remedy is chosen by matching the symptom picture of the patient with that of a remedy. For example, if a person is suffering from diarrhoea and vomiting, minute doses, in potentised form, of a remedy are given which in large, crude doses would cause vomiting and diarrhoea in a healthy person.

Homoeopathic remedies do not work directly on the physical body, but rather, when the healing process is faulty, encourage the natural forces of the body to restore health and harmony. The correct homoeopathic remedy will stimulate the person's vitality to send healing energy where it is needed, i.e. for physical, mental or emotional healing: thus, it is truly a holistic medicine.

The remedies suggested in this book are for use in first-aid and acute situations only. If symptoms are severe, or persist, or are of a more chronic nature, a skilled homoeopath should be consulted. If undergoing a course of homoeopathic treatment from a practitioner, no other remedy should be taken without first consulting them about it. In many cases there is a 'miasmatic' background to an illness, i.e. an acquired or inherited disease tendency; and this can only be dealt with by constitutional treatment from a skilled practitioner.

STORING AND TAKING HOMOEOPATHIC REMEDIES

Homoeopathic remedies are very sensitive and should be stored in a dark, cool place, away from strong smells such as coffee, peppermint, camphor, eucalyptus and menthol. Similarly, those same substances should be avoided by the patient when taking a course of homoeopathic treatment.

Homoeopathic remedies should not be swallowed, but left to dissolve under the tongue. Food, drinks, smoking and toothpaste should be avoided for twenty minutes before and after taking a remedy.

Unless otherwise specified, remedies in the 6th potency should be taken one dose every three hours until there is some improvement, then dosage should be less frequent. Remedies in the 30th potency should only be repeated once or twice, preferably at eight-hour intervals. Remedies in the 200th potency should be taken as a single dose, and not repeated unless otherwise directed. Remedies in any higher potency than the 200th should only be taken under the supervision of a qualified homoeopath.

AROMATHERAPY

Aromatherapy is a form of treatment using essential oils. The term aromatherapy was first used by the French chemist Gattefosse. He researched into the medicinal properties of essential oils in the 1920s. Recorded history of the use of essential oils goes back to the time of the Ancient Egyptians who recognised the effects of fragrant plants, and discovered methods of extracting the oils from the plants to use in perfumes, cooking, ointments and salves and embalming their dead.

Each essential oil has its own therapeutic properties which have been proven by use through the ages, from the Ancient Egyptians, through to the Ancient Greeks, the Arabs, through China and India, and then brought to Europe. Today there is considerable scientific research being done on the properties of the various oils, but we believe that it is the subtle combinations of the components that constitute the whole oil that provides most benefit.

Essential oils are the essences obtained from flowers, leaves, barks, roots and berries by various methods of extraction. The method of extraction used varies according to the type of plant, and the part of the plant to be used. The quality of the oil will depend on the method of extraction and the quality of the plant. Major influences are the area where the plant was grown, and the weather during the growing season, which will be reflected in the price of the oil as with any crop.

Essential oils can be used to treat a wide range of ailments including first-aid, common minor ailments, stress-related diseases and skin problems. They are of great value in skin care, not just for cosmetic purposes, but also to aid such problems as acne, eczema, dermatitis, stretch marks and broken veins. Chemical copies of essential oil fragrances are used widely in commercial cosmetics and perfumery because they are much cheaper; but these will have none of the therapeutic properties of a pure essential oil, and may indeed be damaging if used in therapeutic doses. Check with your supplier that the oils you are going to purchase are pure and unadulterated, and not synthetic or blended oils.

An aromatherapist will use essential oils as part of a holistic programme of treatment. Diet, lifestyle, emotional stress, etc., will all be taken into consideration when choosing appropriate oils to suit the individual. Cleansing diets and exercises may be suggested throughout treatment to enhance healing and relaxation and promote the elimination of toxins. Whilst the oils that we suggest will be helpful to alleviate common and minor ailments, obviously this cannot replace the advice and treatment of a qualified aromatherapist where illness is more persistant or more severe.

HOW TO APPLY ESSENTIAL OILS

Massage

Massage is one of the most successful and effective ways of employing the healing properties of essential oils. There are many good books and courses available today on massage. A regular light massage with essential oils will be beneficial to a person's well-being, and can be relaxing or stimulating depending on the oils chosen.

Before applying essential oils to the skin they must be diluted in a base oil. Suitable vegetable base oils are: almond, apricot kernal, avocado, grapeseed, olive, soya and wheatgerm. Of these, the light oils — almond, apricot kernal, grapeseed, soya — can be used on their own or combined. The heavier oils — avocado, olive, wheatgerm — will be rather strong smelling and sticky if used alone, and are better combined with one of the lighter oils, unless a very rich massage base is required.

The ratio of essential oil to base oil will vary according to the oil and the desired effect, but should fall within the range of one to three per cent of essential oil to base oil. Twenty drops of essential oil equals approximately 1 ml. This means that to 100 ml of base oil between twenty and sixty drops of essential oil (or of combined essential oils) will be added. If you wish to make up enough oil for only one massage then pour a little massage base oil onto a saucer and add just two or three drops of the required essential oil.

Inhalations

Add three or four drops of the essential oil to a handkerchief, hold this near the nose every few moments to inhale the vapours.

Steam inhalations are very effective for congestion and for

treating the skin of the face. To a bowl of steaming water add five to ten drops of essential oil, then place a towel over your head and the bowl and inhale the vapour for a few minutes. This can be repeated two or three times a day.

Baths

In a bath the penetration of the oils into the skin is aided by the heat of the water. Add between five and ten drops of the essential oil to the bath once it has been run and get in the water immediately, before the oils evaporate.

Foot or hand baths may be prepared in the same way using about five drops of essential oil to a bowl of hot water.

Compresses

Compresses can help a wide range of disorders. For a very small area e.g., a boil or insect sting, the essential oil can be used neat. Apply directly to the area and cover with a piece of cotton wool or warm, damp gauze.

For a larger area add ten drops of essential oil to 100 ml of hot water. Soak a piece of clean cotton or lint in the solution and place as hot as possible (without burning the skin) onto the affected area. To keep this warm, place a plastic bag over the cotton and hold a hot water bottle on it.

Scenting a Room

Add ten drops of essential oil to a plant spray containing water and spray in the room to purify the air after cooking, sickness etc.

Aromatic burners can be purchased that use either a nightlight candle or an electric element to heat a plate that a few drops of the oil are placed on.

CAUTION

We do not recommend that essential oils are taken internally although in certain circumstances a qualified aromatherapist may do so.

Essential oils are potentially toxic if used in large doses or if used over a long period of time. Do not use any one oil daily for more than three weeks at a time. Some people may have an adverse reaction to a particular oil, so obviously its use should be discontinued in that case. Use common sense when dealing with these powerful, therapeutic substances.

Oils to be avoided during pregnancy are: basil, camphor, caraway, cedar, chamomile, cinnamon, clary sage, fennel, hyssop, juniper, marjoram, myrrh, nutmeg, oreganum, peppermint, pennyroyal, rosemary, sage, thyme and wintergreen.

Essential oils should never be used on babies. For children oils may be burned in their room or used very well diluted in a massage oil, i.e. do not exceed a one per cent dilution.

Oils made from spices, e.g. black pepper, cinnamon, clove and all the citrus oils can irritate the skin, so do not use unless very well diluted.

We have included a list of aromatherapy books in the Bibliography and we suggest that if you are going to treat yourself or your family with essential oils that you cross-reference any oil we suggest with information on that oil from a more specialist book.

BACH FLOWER REMEDIES®

Bach Flower Remedies are all prepared from the flowers of wild plants, bushes and trees, and none of them are harmful or habit-forming.

They are used, not directly, for physical complaints, but for the sufferer's worry, apprehension, hopelessness, irritability, etc., because these states of mind or moods not only hinder recovery of health and retard convalescence, but are generally accepted as primary causes of sickness and disease.

A long-continued worry or fear, as is well known, will deplete the individual's vitality; he will feel out of sorts, below par, not himself and the body then loses its natural resistance. As peace and harmony is achieved, unity returns to mind and body, closing the circuit as it were and allowing the Life Force to flow freely again, thus providing the body its chance to produce its own natural healing.

This system and the 38 Remedies were discovered by a doctor who had practised for over 20 years in London as a Harley Street consultant, bacteriologist and homoeopath. The late Edward Bach, M.B., B.S., M.R.C.S., L.R.C.P., D.P.H., gave up his lucrative practice in 1930 to devote his full time to seek energies in the plant world which would restore vitality to the sick, so that the sufferer himself would be able to overcome his worry, his apprehension, etc., and so assist in his own healing.

DIRECTIONS

As the Bach Remedies are benign in their action and can result in no unpleasant reactions, they can be taken by anyone. Stock Concentrate Remedies will keep indefinitely — a small size concentrate bottle will provide sufficient to make approximately 45 treatment bottles. More than one Remedy can be taken at the same time — two drops of each chosen Remedy in a cup of water and sipped at intervals, or in a 30 ml (1 fl.oz.) bottle filled with spring water (this represents a treatment bottle) from which four drops are taken directly on the tongue at least four times a day.

It is up to the person to take medical advice if necessary.

RESCUE REMEDY®

Dr Bach combined five specific Remedies from the 38 to formulate an emergency composite that he chose to call 'Rescue Remedy®'. He saved a fisherman's life in 1930 with this preparation.

Its purpose is to comfort/reassure and calm those who have received serious news, severe upset, startling experiences consequently falling into a numbed, bemused state of mind.

To nullify the sufferer's anguish is of the utmost importance in helping the natural healing process of one's being to proceed without hindrance, so the 'Rescue Remedy®' is invaluable to keep at hand for immediate use until the arrival of the doctor if necessary. It does not take the place of medical attention.

'Rescue Remedy®' is taken orally (four drops in water), but can also be applied externally either in liquid or cream form. Animals and plants can also benefit from this treatment.

The information above, and the list in the Appendix, have been printed from the leaflet 'Bach Flower Remedies®', with the kind permission of Bach Flower Remedies® Ltd., Mount Vernon, Sotwell, Wallingford, Oxfordshire OX10 0PZ, UK — the home of Dr Bach where the whole process of making and distributing the Remedies is carried out, and from whom further information and advice is available.

A – Z

of ailments

A

Marshmallow
(Althaea officinalis)

ABRASIONS

A graze: an injury caused by scraping or rubbing. The important thing is to carefully cleanse the area using an antiseptic lotion to prevent infection. A clean, dry dressing may be applied to keep the area protected, this must be changed regularly.

HERBS

Comfrey, Golden Seal, Marigold, St John's Wort: To promote healing and prevent infection.
Combine or use separately. Make an infusion to use as an antiseptic wash, or make a poultice.

Tinctures

Calendula: Promotes healing.
Hypericum: Antiseptic and pain relieving.
You may be able to purchase the above as a mixture referred to as *Hypercal.*
Dilute four or five drops of the tincture in a little cool, boiled water and bathe the area. For a very small area you may apply the tincture neat.

Ointments

Calendula: Promotes healing.
Hypericum: Antiseptic and pain relieving.
You may be able to purchase the above combined in an ointment referred to as *Hypercal Ointment.* Clean the area, then apply the ointment. Cover with a piece of clean lint if required.

HOMOEOPATHY

Arnica 6: To relieve soreness, promote healing and help prevent infection. One dose three times a day for two days.
Ferrum Phos 6X: If there is the suspicion of infection, e.g. heat and redness around the abrased area. One dose three times a day, or crush the tablet and sprinkle the powder directly onto the wound.

AROMATHERAPY

Lavender, Tea Tree: Both these oils have an antiseptic and healing effect. Choose one of them and sprinkle onto the affected area.

ABSCESS

An encapsulated collection of pus. If this becomes inflamed there will be heat, redness and throbbing present.

Anyone who is prone to such infection could benefit from a cleansing diet as well as the following suggestions. Garlic capsules will be a useful dietary supplement. If the patient develops a generalised temperature, or the symptoms are persistant, then professional advice must be sought quickly.

HERBS

External

Chickweed, Comfrey, Marshmallow Root, Plantain, Slippery Elm: Combine or use separately. Make a poultice to draw out the poisons.

Internal

Burdock Root, Chaparral, Cleavers, Echinacea, Golden Seal, Poke Root, Yellow Dock: Combine and make an infusion using one teaspoonful per cup of boiling water. Drink a cupful three times a day for ten days to prevent the infection spreading and eliminate the toxins.

HOMOEOPATHY

Apis 6: Every four hours when there is swelling with stinging pains; there may also be redness and throbbing.
Belladonna 6: Every four hours for a threatening abscess with redness pain and throbbing. The part feels hot to touch.
Calc Sulph 6X: Three times a day if the discharge continues too long and the wound is slow to heal.
Hepar Sulph 6: Three times a day when the pus is forming and it needs to be discharged. The area is very painful and aggravated by touch.
Silica 6X: Three times a day when the pus has formed but the poison is slow to come away. Assists suppuration.

AROMATHERAPY

Chamomile, Lavender: Use externally, making a compress of the neat essential oils.

ACCIDENTS

Most accidents are minor and can be dealt with by using one of the remedies suggested. For more serious accidents, call emergency services and give *Arnica* or *Rescue Remedy*® while waiting. If there is any loss of consciousness or excessive bleeding, seek professional help immediately.

(See also: ABRASIONS, BRUISES, BURNS, EYE INJURIES, FRACTURES, SHOCK, SPRAINS and STRAINS.)

HERBS

Balm, Chamomile, Oats, Scullcap: For shock and stress. Combine or use separately to make a calming infusion. Drink a cupful every few hours as necessary.

HOMOEOPATHY

Arnica for shock and trauma. Reduces pain and bruising and will help prevent haemorrhage.

Arnica 6 or 30: For minor accidents. Take three doses of the 6th potency a day for five days, or one dose of the 30th potency for three days.

Arnica 200: For more severe accidents. Two doses eight hours apart.

Arnica Ointment: This may be applied locally (not for broken skin).

AROMATHERAPY

Eucalyptus, Geranium, Lavender, Tea Tree: These are pain relieving and healing. Apply externally to the affected area.

BACH FLOWER REMEDIES®

Rescue Remedy®*:* For shock and trauma. Take a few drops internally or apply externally.

Rescue Cream®*:* Apply externally.

ACNE

A skin complaint occuring particularly among adolescents. Often this is a result of hormonally induced hyperactivity of the oil-producing glands and is characterised by blackheads and pustules, usually on the face and back.

There is a dietary factor to this condition which is related to the body's ability to metabolise fats and carbohydrates. The intake of fats, sweets and carbohydrates must be reduced and replaced with more fresh fruits and vegetables.

HERBS

Internal

Burdock, Cleavers, Dandelion, Echinacea, Red Clover, Yellow Dock: Combine the herbs and make an infusion using one teaspoon of herbs to one cup of boiling water. Drink a cupful three times a day for at least three weeks. This will help cleanse the system and clear the skin.

External

Chickweed, Elderflower, Marigold: Combine in equal parts and use as a facial steam.

HOMOEOPATHY

For persistant or severe acne constitutional treatment by a qualified practitioner will be necessary.

Silica, Sulphur, Carbo Veg 6X: Cleans out the system, good for unhealthly skin. One three times a day for four days, then two weeks later repeat for four days.

Calc Sulph 6X: For pimples and pustules with a yellow discharge. One twice a day for two weeks.

AROMATHERAPY

Facial steam

Chamomile, Lavender, Petigrain: Add two drops of each oil to hot water and use as a facial steam. Use two or three times a week after cleansing.

Facial oils

Bergamot, Cedarwood, Chamomile, Geranium, Lavender: Dilute in
a suitable vegetable oil base a few drops of the essential oils.
Massage into the skin morning and evening after cleansing.

AGEING

A natural process causing a slowing down of cell division.

Probably the most important factors to consider regarding
ageing are diet, environment and stress. A wholefood diet, with
plenty of fresh fruit and vegetables is vital to provide the right
balance of vitamins and minerals necessary for youthfulness.

The ability to cope with or even enjoy the ageing process
depends on the lifestyle one adopts. Excessive stress is always
ageing and can be rapidly so. Professional counselling can be
very beneficial to help an individual isolate the particular
factors in their lifestyle that could be changed to their long-
term benefit. The following suggestions may be a useful
adjunct to considering appropriate changes in lifestyle.

(See also: WRINKLES.)

HERBS

Comfrey: This herb stimulates healthy cell division. *Comfrey* as
a tea was traditionally drunk on a regular basis to promote
health in old age. As with all medicinal herbs it is advisable
to drink this for a limited period, e.g. twice daily for six
weeks, and not taken indefinitely.

Ginseng: This was traditionally used in China to promote
longevity, aid memory and for its stimulant properties. A
course of *Ginseng* may be taken in a variety of forms, e.g.
root, tincture or tablets, for a month to six weeks of each
year.

HOMOEOPATHY

Calc Phos 6X: Stimulates healthy cell division. Good for exhaustion and for convalescence. Take one dose morning and evening for ten days.

AROMATHERAPY

Lavender: Promotes healthy cell division. Use externally as a massage after diluting in a suitable vegetable oil base. Alternatively add a couple of drops to a warm bath or use as a facial steam.

Neroli, Olibanum, Rose, Sandalwood: A useful combination for ageing skin. Add a few drops of each oil to a suitable vegetable oil base and use as a massage oil. Or combine the oils and use a few drops in a facial steam.

Wheatgerm Oil: This vegetable oil is naturally rich in vitamin E which is said to slow down the ageing process by keeping cells healthy and well oxygenated. Massage the oil into the skin, or take *Wheatgerm Oil* capsules internally; two capsules to be taken three times daily.

ALCOHOLISM

Professional advice should be sought to deal with the physiological and psychological problems related to a dependence on alcohol. One of the most common physical ailments resulting from an excessive intake of alcohol is liver disease. (See also: LIVER PROBLEMS.) The following suggestions are meant to supplement, not replace, professional help.

HERBS

Angelica Root: A cupful drunk on a regular basis is said to create a distaste for alcohol. One cupful three times a day. Not to be taken by diabetics.

Lady's Slipper, Scullcup, Valerian: A tea made from a combination of these herbs will be calming to the nervous system and helpful for withdrawal symptoms including delerium tremens. One cupful three times a day.

HOMOEOPATHY

Individual consultation is recommended.

AROMATHERAPY

A course of treatment by a qualified aromatherapist would be of help to provide support.

BACH FLOWER REMEDIES®

The emotional states leading to a dependence on alcohol are varied. Seek advice or refer to more detailed books on the Bach Flower Remedies®.

ALLERGIES

Allergic reactions are caused when the antigen production of the liver, pancreas and spleen exceed the normal production. Various natural or artificial substances can trigger this response. The most commonly experienced symptoms are irritation of the mucous membranes and skin. A wide range of other symptoms, including behavioural ones, are the subject of extensive recent research.

There are two approaches to the treatment of allergies. One is to isolate the irritating agent and then avoid it, the other is to treat the individual constitutionally until they have a healthier vitality and no longer produce the symptoms of allergy. Professional advice is suggested.

(See also: HAYFEVER.)

HERBS

Chamomile, Yarrow: These herbs will soothe an allergic response. Drink a cupful of the infusion as necessary.

Echinacea, Liquorice, Red Clover: These will help to build up a resistance to allergies. Drink a cupful three times a day for a month. Infuse one heaped teaspoon of the herbs to a cupful of boiling water for ten minutes.

HOMOEOPATHY

Apis 6: Skin allergies with swelling and burning, stinging pains. One three times a day for up to five days.

Ferrum Phos 6X: Will alleviate inflammation or irritation caused by an allergic reaction. One three times a day for up to ten days.

Urtica Urens 6: For alleviation of urticaria, a result of some allergies. One three times a day for up to five days.

AROMATHERAPY

Chamomile, Lavender, Melissa: Apply in a massage oil base for local skin irritation.

BACH FLOWER REMEDIES®

Rescue Cream®: Apply locally to affected area. Good for local skin irritation.

ANAEMIA

Diminished oxygen-carrying capacity of the blood, due to a reduction in the numbers of red cells or in their content of haemoglobin, or both. The cause may be inadequate production of red cells or excessive or prolonged loss of blood. Even a small amount of blood loss over a prolonged period of time may cause anaemia, e.g. from an internal ulcer, so persistent

9

anaemia should always be referred to a practitioner for precise diagnosis.

Many women are considered to be anaemic due to an inability to assimilate iron at a rate sufficient to make up for that lost in the blood during the menstrual cycle.

Laxatives will cause a loss of iron from the body, and continual drinking of coffee and tea will retard the absorption of the mineral iron. Many drugs will also cause anaemia.

The mineral iron is essential for the formation of red blood cells. Foods naturally rich in iron include: meat, eggs, lentils, apricots, green-leaf vegetables, molasses and beetroot.

The minerals calcium and copper, vitamin C and the B group vitamins must also be present for the body to be able to assimilate iron. A balanced diet of natural foods should supply sufficient quantities of these vitamins and minerals, otherwise food supplements may be taken, and vegetarians in particular may require additional vitamin B12.

HERBS

Alfalfa, Centaury, Dandelion Root, Nettle, Rosehip, Watercress, Yellow Dock: Combine and make an infusion using one teaspoon of herbs to a cup of boiling water. Drink a cupful three times a day for a month to six weeks.

HOMOEOPATHY

For chronic cases, a qualified homoeopath should be consulted.

Ferrum Phos 6X and Kali Sulph 6X: These two tissue salts taken in combination will enable the body to assimilate iron and use it more efficiently. Take one *Ferrum Phos* in the morning and one *Kali Sulph* at bedtime for three weeks.

BACH FLOWER REMEDIES®

Olive: This will help with the exhaustion and weariness often associated with anaemia.

ANOREXIA NERVOSA

This is a disease usually occuring in adolescent girls. The obsessive desire to diet, to lose real or imagined excess weight, results in the sufferer becoming progressively less able to eat any food. Occasional binging (frantic overeating) may occur.

Amenorrhoea (absent periods) is a common symptom. Severe cases of anorexia nervosa can be fatal.

Professional help is essential, and the following suggestions are only to be taken as an adjunct to treatment from a practitioner, and with their approval.

(See also: APPETITE LOSS.)

HERBS

Balm, Centaury, Dandelion, Liquorice, Vervain: These herbs may help to stimulate the appetite, and are relaxing. Combine and make an infusion using one heaped teaspoon of herbs to one cupful of boiling water and stand for ten minutes. Drink a cupful three times a day for up to one month.

HOMOEOPATHY

Avena Sativa Tincture: Helps underlying anxiety and stimulates the appetite. Five drops in a wine glass of water three times a day.

Calc Phos 6X: Assists healthy digestion and assimilation of food. Good for the convalescent stage of any disease; helps to stimulate the appetite. One dose three times a day for two weeks.

AROMATHERAPY

Bergamot, Clary Sage, Rose. A regular bath or massage with these oils may be of benefit.

BACH FLOWER REMEDIES®

Consult books on the Bach Flower Remedies® for more detailed information or visit a professional prescriber.

11

ANXIETY

A feeling of uneasiness and apprehension accompanied with tension which may or may not have an obvious cause. Anxiety may be associated with tight breathing, palpitations and perspiration.

Continued anxiety can cause illness such as digestive disorders, headaches, backache, high blood pressure and many other troubles.

Counselling may be needed to help the person redirect their fears and understand their symptoms. A professional practitioner should be consulted if the anxiety is extreme.

Diet, as always, has an important role to play. Check especially that your diet contains sufficient calcium and magnesium, and vitamins B and C.

HERBS

Balm, Catnip, Chamomile, Hops, Lime Flowers, Orange Blossom, Passiflora, Scullcap, Valerian, Vervain, Wood Betony: These are all relaxing nervines. Select from these herbs to make a mixture. Combine and drink a cupful of infusion three times a day.

HOMOEOPATHY

AAA 6: (Ambra Grisea, Anacardium, Arg Nit) Anxiety prior to a particular event, e.g. aeroplane flight, interview, exam, etc. Take one dose a week before the event and one dose three times on the day.

Arg Nit 30: Anticipatory diarrhoea. Stage fright, etc. One or two doses.

Calc Phos, Kali Phos, Mag Phos 6X: Nervous fatigue. Calms down after stress and strain. Results of work pressure. Stress headaches. Inability to relax. One three times a day for ten days or when necessary.

12

Calc Phos, Kali Phos, Nat Phos 6X: Students preparing for exams, suffering from over-studying and anxiety. One three times a day for ten days.

Ignatia 200: Anxiety dating from a particular disappointment, shock, bereavement, etc. One dose.

Kali Phos 6X: Nervousness, sleeplessness, weariness, tension. For nerves 'on edge'. One three times a day for ten days.

Mag Phos 6X: Nervous tension and tense muscles causing cramps, headaches, trembling, etc. One three times a day for ten days.

AROMATHERAPY

Basil, Geranium, Lavender, Melissa, Rose: Add two or three drops to a bath, or combine two or three and dilute in a suitable base massage oil for a relaxing massage. As a soothing fragrance *Basil* and *Clary Sage* could be used on an aromatic burner.

BACH FLOWER REMEDIES®

Choose from among the following and refer to a more detailed book to see if there are indications for other Bach Flower Remedies®.

Rescue Remedy®: Apprehension, shock, anguish, panic attacks, etc.

Agrimony: For those who suffer anxiety but pretend to be happy and cheerful.

Aspen: Vague anxiety, apprehensions and fears of unknown origin.

Cherry Plum: Desperation, fear of mental collapse.

Mimulus: Fear and apprehension of known events.

Red Chestnut: Anxiety about others, e.g. members of one's family.

Rock Rose: Extreme anxiety, panic.

White Chestnut: Persistent anxious thoughts. Preoccupation with some worry.

13

APHRODISIACS

An agent which increases sexual desire and improves sexual potency.

HERBS

Damiana, Saw Palmetto: Hormonal tonics for the male reproductive system; traditionally used as sexual stimulants. Combine and drink three times daily using one teaspoonful of herb per cupful of boiling water, standing for ten minutes.
Ginseng: A traditional aphrodisiac if taken on a regular basis, e.g., daily for a month. Use as root, tincture or tablets.
False Unicorn: Stimulates the female hormonal system. Make a decoction and drink twice a day for a month.

HOMOEOPATHY

Constitutional treatment to build up the vitality is recommended.

AROMATHERAPY

Clary Sage, Jasmine, Patchouli, Rose, Sandalwood, Ylang Ylang: Combine two or three of these essential oils and mix into a vegetable base oil for a sexually stimulating massage, or add two or three drops of one of the essential oils to a warm bath. Alternatively, a few drops of one of the oils burnt in an essential oil burner will create a suitably relaxing atmosphere.

APPETITE LOSS

The appetite can be a good indicator of the general state of health. Chronic appetite loss should be referred to a practitioner.

The remedies suggested here will be useful in the recovery phase of an illness such as influenza.

(See also: ANOREXIA NERVOSA, CONVALESCENCE.)

HERBS

Centaury, Gentian, Hops, Wormwood: These 'bitter' herbs will stimulate the appetite. Combine the herbs and make an infusion, drink three times a day. Alternatively take in tincture form.

HOMOEOPATHY

Calc Phos 6X: Assists digestion and assimilation of food. Good for convalescence, may help stimulate the appetite. Take one twice a day for ten days.

AROMATHERAPY

Bergamot, Coriander, Fennel, Juniper: Dilute in a vegetable base oil and rub into the stomach area twice daily to help stimulate the appetite.

ARTHRITIS

Inflammation of a joint, causing pain and leading to restriction of movement. A holistic style practitioner should be consulted because it is essential to treat the whole being; otherwise healing will be only slight or temporary. Factors that need to be investigated are: the genetic framework, environmental factors — diet, stress, injury — and also the pyschological contribution.

The most common forms of this disease are osteo-arthritis and rheumatoid arthritis.

Again, it must be stressed that professional guidance is essential; the following suggestions may provide some relief whilst professional help is being sought. Acupuncture and naturopathy are particularly recommended for this complaint.

(See also: GOUT, RHEUMATISM.)

HERBS

Ash, Celery Seed, Cornsilk, Devil's Claw, Feverfew, Meadowsweet, Prickly Ash, White Willow: A mixture to clear uric acid and

15

toxins, reduce inflammation and relieve pain.

Add *Bogbean* if the symptoms are worse in damp weather.

Combine the herbs and drink an infusion three times daily for one month to six weeks.

A poultice for swollen joints that are relieved by warmth may be made from nine parts of *Slippery Elm* to one part of *Cayenne*. Add 75 g of the mixture to hot water to make a paste. Spread onto a cloth and apply to the affected area. Leave on for as long as possible.

Alternatively, for joints that are relieved by cool, a cabbage poultice will be helpful.

HOMOEOPATHY

Constitutional treatment will be of most benefit. The following may assist while alternative treatment is being considered.

Apis, Benz Ac, Ledum 6X: Swollen, painful joints. Pain alleviated by cold bathing. Dissolves acid deposits. One twice a day for ten days.

Ferrum Phos 6X: In acute attacks with inflammation of the joint. One three times a day for up to ten days.

Nat Phos 6X: Will help clear out uric acid. One twice a day for ten days.

AROMATHERAPY

Chamomile, Eucalyptus, Juniper, Lavender, Lemon: Combine and dilute in almond oil, massage into the afflicted joint and wrap in a warm cover. Or add a few drops of the chosen essential oil or oils to a warm bath.

FOOD SUPPLEMENTS

Cider Vinegar, Honey: Add a teaspoon of each to a cupful of hot water. Drink at least every morning, and preferably three times a day.

Cod Liver Oil Capsules: Two capsules three times a day.

The diet should be checked for an adequate supply of vitamins B and C

ASTHMA

Asthma can be defined as a difficulty in breathing caused by muscular spasm. The spasm makes it difficult to cough away mucous which collects in the small bronchi thus further impeding breathing.

There is a hereditary factor to asthma, and other causes include allergy, infection and emotional disturbance. Treatment of asthma is a difficult, complicated problem and should be handled by a qualified practitioner. In particular, the assessment of the severity of acute episodes calls for considerable experience.

A diet eliminating all mucous-stimulating foods (e.g. dairy products) may be of help.

The switch over from orthodox inhalers and medication should not be attempted unless under the supervision of a suitably qualified practitioner. The following suggestions may offer some relief whilst such professional help is being sought.

HERBS

Elecampane, Wild Cherry Bark: Help to strengthen the lungs. Infuse one teaspoonful of herbs to a cupful of boiling water for ten minutes. Strain and drink a cupful twice a day for ten days.

Coltsfoot, Comfrey, Elecampane, Grindelia, Heartsease, Hyssop, Liquorice, Mullein: An expectorant mixture to help clear mucous and tonify the lungs. Mix in equal parts. Infuse one teaspoonful of herbs to a cupful of boiling water for ten minutes. Drink a cupful three times a day for up to a month.

Motherwort, Scullcap: A soothing and calming mixture to drink after a spasm attack. Combine and drink a cupful of the infusion every couple of hours.

17

HOMOEOPATHY

Constitutional treatment by a qualified practitioner can be of great benefit to asthma sufferers.

Mag Phos 6X: May help to relax spasms. Take one dose every two hours during an attack, or one dose three times a day for ten days as a longer-term course.

AROMATHERAPY

Chamomile, Eucalyptus, Hyssop, Lavender: Add two drops of each of the essential oils to a bowl of hot water and inhale the vapour.

BACH FLOWER REMEDIES®

Rescue Remedy®: Add a few drops to a little water and sip as often as required to alleviate fear and panic.

ATHLETE'S FOOT

A fungal infection of the skin, usually found between the toes.
  Keep the feet clean and dry. Wear only natural fibres for socks and shoes. If the toes are pushed together place a small piece of cotton wool between them so that air can circulate and moisture is not retained.

Calendula Talc: Can be used after bathing to heal the skin and absorb moisture.

HERBS

Burdock, Heartsease, Thyme, Yellow Dock: Combine and make an infusion to drink three times a day for at least two weeks.

Marigold, Myrrh, Thyme: Combine the tinctures or make an infusion to bathe the affected part three times a day.

HOMOEOPATHY

Nat Phos, Nat Sulph, Silica 6X: For fungal infections. One three times a day for ten days.

Calendula Tincture: Apply regularly on cotton wool to help dry up the fungus and heal the skin.

AROMATHERAPY

Eucalyptus, Lavender, Pine, Thyme: Combine the above oils and make a strong dilution in a vegetable oil base. Massage a couple of drops of the oil into the affected area twice a day after bathing.

Tea Tree: Apply directly to the affected area.

B

Mountain Tobacco~(Arnica Montana)

BACKACHE

Pains in the back are experienced by many people and the causes are very varied. Bad posture caused by tension will create strained muscles resulting in pain. We would advise the Alexander Technique to correct this. Pain in the back at the level of the waist may be due to spinal disease, or kidney and bladder infections; various toxins otherwise eliminated through the kidney and bladder are deposited in surrounding tissue areas, especially the spinal joints of the lumbar region. Low back pain may be due to a disorder of the reproductive organs in women. Much back pain is the result of overstraining or injury. If the vertebra or pelvis is out of alignment, a manipulative therapy such as Osteopathy or Chiropractice should be considered. A diagnosis to rule out a more serious causative factor is vital: full examination, X-rays, or other investigations may be indicated.

HERBS

Buchu, Cornsilk, Couchgrass, Nettle, Uva Ursi: Are cleansing and de-toxifying herbs for the lower back area. Combine equal parts and infuse one teaspoon in a cupful of boiling water. Drink two times a day for three weeks.
Balm, Lady's Slipper, Vervain, White Willow: For inflammation

20

and pain. Combine and infuse one teaspoon of equal parts of the herbs to drink when necessary.

Comfrey Oil: Massage daily.

HOMOEOPATHY

Arnica 6 or 30: Take three doses of the 6th potency a day for five days, or one dose of the 30th potency a day for three days. When pain is after an accident or from over-exertion such as gardening, dancing or playing sports.

Hypericum 30 or 200: One or two doses for injuries involving the spinal nerves. Backache resulting from spinal injury in the past, pain in the coccycx after childbirth.

Mag Phos 6X: One three times a day for up to ten days for neuralgic pains along the spine, muscle tension and spasm, sharp shooting pains relieved by warmth.

Rhus Tox 6 or 30: Take three doses of the 6th potency twice a day for five days, or one dose of the 30th potency for three days. For muscular stiffness due to over-exertion or from exposure to cold and damp.

AROMATHERAPY

Celery, Ginger, Juniper, Marjoram, Parsley, Sage: For a soothing and warming massage. Combine five drops of each in a light vegetable oil base and massage over the painful area.

BED WETTING

This is not usually considered a problem until the child reaches school age. It is very often hereditary, and sometimes caused by an organic problem, so it is advisable to take the child to a physician for an examination. There is nearly always a psychological factor to take into account. Prolonged bed wetting causes stress to the child and to the parents, so it must be treated with care and understanding. A non-stimulating diet

should be encouraged cutting out soft drinks, white sugar, and food colourings, especially orange.
(See also: INCONTINENCE.)

HERBS

Catnip, Chamomile, Horsetail, St John's Wort: Use one teaspoon to a cup and sweeten with a little buckwheat honey so the child will drink it. Try two cups a day.

HOMOEOPATHY

There are numerous remedies to help in this situation and it is important to find the correct remedy that fits the nature of the child, so if the pattern persists or the child suddenly starts wetting the bed, go and see a homoeopath.

BACH FLOWER REMEDIES®

Look at the remedies covering fears and anxiety and decide if your child could be helped by them. (See the list in the Appendix and cross-reference with more detailed books mentioned in the Bibliography.)

BITES AND STINGS

Some people are more sensitive than others to bites. If symptoms of collapse or difficulty in breathing develop, emergency professional treatment must be sought. The following remedies will help deal with the pain, sting or shock; but it is also important to employ methods to stop infection developing.

HERBS

Marshmallow, Witchazel: To help with bruising and swelling. Make an infusion and apply externally.
Marigold, St John's Wort: If the skin is broken, to prevent

infection and promote healing. Make an infusion and apply externally at regular intervals.

To prevent a bite becoming infected take *Echinacea* decoction or tincture internally. Crushed *Garlic* or a slice of raw *Onion* applied externally may relieve stinging and reduce risk of infection.

Lavender, Pennyroyal, Pyrethrum, Southernwood, Tansy, Wormwood: For repelling insects. Make an infusion from the above herbs and apply to the skin (when cool), or spray in a room.

HOMOEOPATHY

Apis 6 or 30: Wasp or bee stings, swelling, redness, stinging, smarting pains, worse for heat. Symptoms of collapse. One every few hours until improvement occurs.

Arnica 30: Bites from mammals where bruising is marked and shock is present. One or two doses.

Caladium 6 or 30: Mosquito bites. Either take as a prophylactic, or after exposure. Two or three times a day as necessary.

Hypericum 30: Punctured skin by bites or stings; skin tingling, burning pains radiating from injury. One or two doses.

Lachesis 30: Bites from poisonous animals, e.g. snakes, spiders. Part looks purple or blue. This is only a temporary measure on your way to the emergency room at the hospital.

Ledum 6 or 30: Punctured wounds, dog or insect bites. Oedematous swelling, bruising, parts can become red and inflamed. Bites may become infected. Try this remedy first for horsefly, wasp and dog bites. One dose as often as needed.

External

Hypericum Tincture, Ledum, Pyrethrum, Rumex: These can be bought in combination and used as an anti-sting lotion — dilute and apply locally before exposure or when bitten.

Hypercal Tincture: Apply to bites and stings to soothe and help prevent infection.

AROMATHERAPY

Citronella, Lemon Grass, Peppermint: Use diluted in vegetable oil as a repellant, apply to exposed areas. We recommend also

23

that these oils can be burned in the room to deter insects.

Eucalyptus, Lavender, Melissa: After-sting care. Dab any of these oils on the affected area.

Tea Tree: This can be used neat as a repellant and to relieve a bite or sting.

BACH FLOWER REMEDIES®

Rescue Remedy®: To soothe the patient and help with shock. Take a few drops internally or apply externally.

Rescue Cream®: Apply locally to soothe the bite or sting.

BOILS

A boil is a painful, acute inflammation around the root of a hair.

Boils must not be squeezed as this would cause infection to spread. Boils are a symptom that the body contains waste and toxic matter, so a cleansing diet is recommended along with appropriate treatment.

HERBS

Marshmallow, Slippery Elm: Use either herb as a poultice to help draw pus from the boil.

Echinacea, Poke Root: A blood purifying combination. Combine in equal parts and make a decoction using a heaped teaspoon of herbs to a mug of water and simmer for ten minutes. Strain and drink a cupful three times a day for ten days. These herbs may be taken as tinctures: combine and take a teaspoonful in a cup of warm water three times a day for ten days.

HOMOEOPATHY

Arnica 6: A crop of small, painful boils. One dose three times a day for five days.

Belladonna 6: The boil is beginning to form. Heat, throbbing pain and redness are present. One dose three times a day for three days.

Gunpowder 3x: A homoeopathic blood cleanser. Take one dose three times a day for ten days.

Silica 6X: For boils where the pus has formed but healing has come to a standstill. One dose three times a day for up to five days.

Tarentula 6: Boils that are very painful and inflamed: intense itching and burning pains. One dose three times a day for up to five days.

AROMATHERAPY

Chamomile, Lavender, Lemon, Thyme: Any of the above may be used. Add two or three drops to half a cupful of warm water; dip in a piece of cotton wool and apply this to the boil. Repeat two or three times a day.

BREAST FEEDING

All indications suggest that the breast-fed child will be healthier; the colostrum produced after childbirth contains antibodies which give protection against infections. This early protection fills the immunity gap and so babies fed on breast milk are more resistant to infections than those fed by bottled milk. Putting the baby to the breast as soon as the cord is cut encourages the flow of milk, gives comfort to the baby and forms an early bond with the mother. Breast feeding is usually on demand, which means it is going to be draining for the mother, so plenty of rest is needed between feeds. Small regular meals and an increase in fluids are needed to help maintain a flow of milk, avoid over-spiced foods, garlic and acid fruits which might cause colic in the baby.
(See also: MASTITIS.)

HERBS

Aniseed, Borage, Caraway, Fennel, Fenugreek, Holy thistle: To maintain sufficient supply of milk. Combine and infuse one teaspoon to a cupful of boiling water, and drink two or three times daily.

Alfalfa is rich in minerals and *Vervain* is soothing, so these can be drunk when needed as an infusion.

If it becomes necessary to dry up the milk, drink an infusion of *Sage* three times a day.

Comfrey Ointment: This may be applied externally to heal cracked nipples.

HOMOEOPATHY

Calc Phos 6X: Three times a day for maintaining general health. Exhaustion.

Calendula Tincture: For cracked painful nipples; bathe with ten drops diluted in warm water.

Causticum 6: Three times a day for cracked nipples and poor milk flow.

China 6: Twice daily for exhaustion brought on by breast feeding. Take for ten days.

Silica 6X: Three times a day for two days if there is any sign of abscess forming on the nipple, reducing the flow of milk.

These homoeopathic suggestions can be tried, but do consult a homoeopath if the symptoms persist for longer than two days.

AROMATHERAPY

Rose: For sore nipples; massage with a couple of drops of Rose oil in a little almond oil base. Wash before feeding, as any essential oils are too strong for the baby.

Geranium, Lavender, Rose: For inflammation of the breast, dilute one drop of each in a pint of cold water and use as a compress. However, if the condition persists, consult a practitioner.

BACH FLOWER REMEDIES®

Olive: This might be useful for the extreme exhaustion felt by some nursing mothers.

BRONCHITIS

Acute bronchitis is a common condition involving inflammation and infection of the respiratory tract. It is common in the winter months and particularly in the elderly, the frail and those with a chronic chest disorder. Acute bronchitis often occurs in children with infectious fevers, especially measles, influenza and whooping cough. Symptoms are those of a mild fever with a cough, possibly pain beneath the sternum and breathing is usually a little faster than normal. The condition usually subsides in a few days with rest in bed, and is serious only in young children and elderly people where inflammation may spread and cause broncho-pneumonia. Repeated attacks may give rise to chronic bronchitis.

In chronic bronchitis there is swelling and thickening of the lining of the bronchial tree and obstruction to air entry is made worse by the presence of thick mucous. This can cause a serious debility, and must be dealt with by an experienced practitioner. Cigarette smoking, air pollution by smoke and sulphur dioxide, or working in a dusty atmosphere may be contributing causes.

Chronic bronchitis must be referred to a practitioner for constitutional treatment. The following remedies may be tried for the early stages of acute bronchitis, but in young children or if the symptoms persist then professional help should be sought.

HERBS

Aniseed, Coltsfoot, Elecampane, Hyssop, Iceland Moss, Lungwort, Wild Cherry Bark: These herbs combine an expectorant effect with a demulcent action, soothing the inflamed tissues.

27

Combine and infuse one teaspoon to a cup three times a day.

HOMOEOPATHY

Aconite 6 or 30: Take three doses of the 6th potency a day for five days, or one dose of the 30th potency a day for three days. When cough comes on suddenly after exposure to cold winds, beginning of a fever, short dry cough which wakes the patient from sleep, patient is frightened and restless.

Ant Tart 6 or 30: Two or three doses for three or four days, patient is pale with a cold sweat, rattling cough with much mucous in the chest but less and less is raised as the patient becomes weaker. Coated tongue, averse to food and drink.

Ars Alb 6 or 30; Two or three doses for three or four days, suffocative cough, great tightness felt in the chest. Patient is frightened, anxious and restless, chilly patient. Desires sips of hot drinks.

Belladonna 6 or 30: Two or three doses for two or three days, for spasmodic cough with fever. Patient is delirious and has a high fever.

Bryonia 6 or 30: Two or three doses a day for three or four days for hard, dry, barking cough. Chest is painful and patient holds it when coughing, cough worse at night and from eating and drinking. Very irritable patient who wants to be left alone. Thirsty.

Causticum 6 or 30: Two or three doses for three or four days for a hard, scraping cough which hurts the chest. Any mucous slips back down before it can be cleared.

Ferrum Phos 6X: Three times a day for three or four days for the first signs of fever and inflammation. Short, acute, painful coughs. Try this first and hopefully other remedies won't be needed if you act fast enough.

Ipecac 6 or 30: Two or three doses over two or three days when the cough is preceeded by vomiting or mucous causes vomiting. Useful in children who cannot raise the mucous by coughing, but do vomit it up.

Phosphorus 6 or 30: Two or three doses for three or four days with a very irritating, tormenting cough, thirst for ice cold drinks, patient is shaking and weak, fearful and does not want to be left alone.

Pulsatilla 6 or 30: Two or three doses over three or four days with a catarrhal condition which descends to the chest; may follow on from measles. Thick yellow-green catarrh, tightness in chest, desires fresh air, dry cough worse at night.

Sulphur 30: Two or three doses eight hours apart when there is a sensation of weight on the chest, unpleasant smelling sweat, waves of heat and cold, patient is weary and not responding well to treatment, red orifices.

AROMATHERAPY

Benzoin, Eucalyptus, Thyme: Inhale steam from a bowl of hot water into which two or three drops of the essential oil has been put, or dilute in a vegetable base oil to massage onto the chest area.

BRUISES

A bruise is the result of a blow or fall causing damage to the soft tissue beneath the skin, breaking the skin capillaries. As the blood clots the bruise becomes discoloured.

HERBS

Comfrey, Marigold, Witchazel, Yarrow: Make an infusion using one tablespoon of each to a pint of water and use as a compress over the injured area.

Arnica Ointment: This is the most effective remedy for bruises but do not use if the skin is broken.

Arnica Tincture: This can also be used. Apply externally.

Witchazel distilled: Dab on locally with cotton wool.

HOMOEOPATHY

Arnica 6 or 30: Take one three times a day to help the bruising and to counteract any effects of shock. Take for two days.
Hypericum 6 or 30: Two doses where bruising is very painful and relieved by warmth.
Ledum 6 or 30: Two doses when bruising becomes black or swollen, e.g. black eyes.
Ruta 6 or 30: Two doses for painful bruising of the bones e.g. shin.

AROMATHERAPY

Lavender: Apply locally over bruised area.
Hyssop, Marigold (Tagetes), Marjoram: Dilute in cold water and use as a compress.

BACH FLOWER REMEDIES®

Rescue Cream®: Apply locally.
Rescue Remedy®: Use internally where shock is involved. Take a few drops as required.

BURNS

Treatment obviously depends on the severity of the burn; minor burns and scalds can be dealt with safely at home, more serious burns should be admitted to casualty, without attempting to remove clothing, etc., which may further damage the skin. Internal treatment for shock, e.g. *Rescue Remedy®* may safely be given. Chemical burns must be washed with cold running water for at least five minutes. If blisters form do not puncture as they form a protective cushion to the damaged area.

HERBS

Aloe Vera: An excellent remedy for burns, including sunburn. Grow a plant in the kitchen, break off a leaf and squeeze out the gel on the burn. It is also available commercially as an ointment or gel.

Comfrey, Marigold, St John's Wort: Make an infusion from any of the above and bathe the burn to help promote healing.

Tinctures

When using tinctures to treat burns add a teaspoonful of tincture to a cupful of cool, boiled water. Soak a pad of gauze in this lotion, which must be large enough to cover the burn, apply the gauze, cover with lint and bandage. Remove the lint whenever the dressing feels dry and resoak the gauze by moistening it with a few drops of the lotion, this prevents any tearing of the new skin cells and allows undisturbed growth to take place under cover of the dressing. Once a scab begins to form the burn should be kept as dry as possible.

Hypericum: For deeper burns and scalds, also for burns which are becoming infected due to mistreatment. Apply as directed.

Urtica Urens: For simple burns and scalds, use as directed or sprinkle undiluted over a minor burn which can then be left open to the atmosphere.

Ointments

Useful for soothing minor burns and scalds. Apply liberally over the affected area as soon as possible. Either cover with a light dressing or leave exposed to the atmosphere.

Hypericum and Urtica: Apply locally to the affected area.

HOMOEOPATHY

Cantharis 30: One or two doses a day for two to three days. Burns and scalds with stinging, smarting pains where blistering is predominant.

Causticum 30: One or two doses a day for two to three days. Severe and painful burns.

Kali Bich 200: Two doses twelve hours apart for severe pains in deep burns and old burn scarring.

31

Urtica Urens 6 or 30: Two or three doses over two to three days for simple, non-severe burns and scalds.

AROMATHERAPY

Lavender: Used undiluted will soothe a burn, prevent infection, and help promote new tissue growth. The fragrance will also be useful for the trembling or panic that may accompany the burn. Apply liberally onto the affected area.

BACH FLOWER REMEDIES®

Rescue Cream®: Apply locally to the affected area.

C

Frankincense
(Olibanum)

CATARRH

Inflammation of the sensitive mucous membrane lining of nasal passages, throat and sinuses leads to an increased production of mucous, which in the healthy state is secreted to moisten and protect the area.

This may become a chronic problem, recurring each winter, in which case professional advice should be sought. There is a hereditary factor. For catarrh and congestion following a cold the suggested remedies below may be tried.

Diet is an important consideration; milk and all dairy products should be eliminated from the diet. Plenty of salads, vegetables, fresh fruits, garlic and onions need to be included. (See also: SINUSITIS.)

HERBS

Bayberry, Elderflower, Eyebright, Golden Rod, Plantain: These are anti-catarrhal and will bring relief. Combine and drink three times a day for two to three weeks.

Echinacea: This may be added if infection is involved.

Golden Seal: This may be added to the mixture but should be used with some discretion, for although it is extremely effective, some people find that it has a drying effect on the mucous membranes if use is prolonged.

HOMOEOPATHY

In cases of chronic catarrh, professional advice should be sought, as there is often a miasmatic (inherited or acquired through suppression) background to this problem. For short-term relief the following may be helpful:

Bryonia 6: Take one three times a day for up to five days, for catarrh accompanied by offensive smell and coughing up of mucous. Headache with 'stuffed up' sensation.

Calc Sulph 6X: Thick, blood-streaked discharge of mucous. Three times a day for five days.

Calc Sulph, Kali Sulph, Nat Sulph 6X: For blocked sinuses and stuffed up sensation at the end of a cold. One three times a day for up to ten days.

Hepar Sulph 6: Thick yellow mucous with painful inflammation at the root of the nose. Worse in cold, dry wind. One three times a day for up to five days.

Kali Bich 6: Tough stringy plugs of mucous. Pain in the sinuses and at the root of the nose. Take one three times a day, for up to five days.

Kali Mur 6X: Thick, white, bland catarrh; stuffed up sensation of nose and ears. Three times a day for five to ten days.

Kali Sulph 6X: Yellow, slimy discharge of mucous from the nose; symptoms worse in the evenings and in warm rooms; longing for fresh air. Three times daily for five to ten days.

Nat Mur 6X: Watery discharge from nose and watering eyes. Sense of smell lost, much sneezing. One three times a day for up to ten days.

Silica 6X: Yellow-green nasal discharge with tendency to nose bleeds. Dry hard crusts in nose. Take one three times a day, for up to ten days.

AROMATHERAPY

Eucalyptus, Frankincense (Olibanum), Peppermint, Pine: Add two to three drops of the essential oils to a steam inhalation, or to a vegetable oil base, e.g. almond oil and rub onto the chest.

CELLULITE

Cellulite is formed when the fat cells become interspersed with water and skin feels uneven and bumpy. Cellulite usually appears on the thighs, buttocks, and hips although it may appear virtually anywhere on the body.

Cellulite seems to be hormonally related and thus mild forms of it occur during different times of the menstrual cycle, or at times of hormonal upheaval such as pregnancy or the menopause. Use of the birth control pill might aggravate it. Bad circulation may also be a cause, therefore taking exercise and giving up smoking will help. In order to increase the circulation, try massaging with a body brush or a loofah.

Certain foods provoke fluid retention, and aggravate the cellulite problem, so treatment should include the avoidance of smoked or salty foods, sugar and refined carbohydrates.

HERBS

Agnus, Castus, Ash, Birch, Cascara Sagrada, Cayenne Pepper, Dandelion, Fennel, Poke Root, Red Clover, Yellow Dock: These herbs will gently cleanse the lymphatic system, have a mildly diuretic effect and rebalance the hormones. Combine the herbs, make an infusion, and drink three times daily for six weeks.

HOMOEOPATHY

In order to get to the root of the problem, constitutional treatment will be necessary. The following tissue salts may be of help.

Nat Phos 6X: Regulates the distribution of intercellular fluids, most useful when acid conditions, e.g. rheumatism, digestive upsets or liver problems are found in association with cellulite. One twice daily for ten days.

Nat Sulph 6X: The excess water eliminator. Also helps clear out toxic fluids. Liverish symptoms may be present. One twice daily for ten days.

AROMATHERAPY

Black Pepper, Cypress, Fennel, Juniper, Lemon: These help to eliminate toxins and disperse water. Add a few drops of each

35

to a vegetable oil base, massage in morning and night, and also after a bath or sauna.

CHICKENPOX (VARICELLA)

Chickenpox is one of the most contagious of all the childhood illnesses. The contagious period is from 24 hours before the rash starts to the time they scab over. Chickenpox may begin with a temperature, but often a rash is the first sign; this will appear in different parts of the body and will be extremely itchy. At first the spots are like dark red pimples; within a couple of hours they will have developed a small blister on top which resembles a drop of water, this will eventually form a scab and drop off.

Chickenpox is nearly always a mild disease, the most frequent complication being infection of the rash through scratching. As with all self-limiting childhood diseases it is important not to suppress the symptoms no matter what. Acute illness should be seen as an opportunity for the vitality to assert itself and throw off inherited or acquired toxicity.

HERBS

Internal

Balm, Burdock, Echinacea, Elderflower, Heartsease: Combine and drink an infusion three times daily, to soothe the patient and encourage rapid recovery. *Chamomile* and *Scullcap* will be useful if there is anxiety or restlessness present.

External

Chickweed, Lavender, Marigold, St John's Wort: These may be combined to make a soothing and healing lotion, infuse, cool, and apply regularly with cotton wool.
Sponge the body with diluted *Witchazel* to cool and relieve irritation if needed.

Comfrey Ointment: This may be massaged in once the pustules have stopped forming and the scabs have fallen off, to prevent scarring and promote skin healing.

Stellaria Ointment: Soothing and cooling for the rash. Apply locally.

HOMOEOPATHY

Ant Crud 6 or 30: For a child who is irritable and does not want to be touched. Fearful itching worse when warm in bed.

Ant Tart 6 or 30: Skin eruption develops slowly. Rash accompanied by a rattling cough or bronchitis.

Ars Alb 6 or 30: Large pus-filled eruptions, which may become open sores, burning pains accompany extreme chilliness. The patient is very restless and anxious.

Belladonna 6 or 30: For symptoms of fever, and red itching skin. Take three doses of the 6th potency a day for five days, or one dose of the 30th potency a day for three days.

Pulsatilla 6 or 30: For a weepy child, who is not thirsty despite fever. Take three doses of the 6th potency a day for five days, or one dose of the 30th potency a day for three days.

Rhus Tox 6 or 30: Eruptions which burn and itch, restlessness during the night. Take three doses of the 6th potency a day for five days, or one dose of the 30th potency a day for three days. This is the main remedy to ease discomfort and itching.

Variolinum 30: For a stubborn case of chickenpox, that is not responding well to treatment, or is dragging on too long. Give only two doses twelve hours apart.

AROMATHERAPY

Chamomile, Lavender, Tea Tree: Add a few drops of each to a vegetable base oil and rub into the body for a soothing and healing effect.

CHILBLAINS

These occur due to an inadequate supply of blood to the extremeties, i.e. fingers and toes, causing swelling, itching and burning sensations. A combination of treatment will be necessary to eradicate and prevent chilblains as several factors are involved. Locally, extremes of temperature should be avoided, well-fitting shoes should be worn with natural fibres next to the skin, applications to ease itching and soreness may be used. To assist circulation, constitutional treatment by a holistic practitioner is recommended. Diet is an important factor; salty foods and animal fats should be avoided. Foods rich in rutin, e.g. buckwheat, or rutin tablets will help strengthen the blood vessels and improve the circulation.

HERBS

Internal

Buckwheat, Ginger, Hawthorn, Prickly Ash: Combined with a pinch of *Cayenne*, these will stimulate the circulation. Make an infusion and drink a cupful three times daily for six weeks.

External

Calendula, Myrrh, Witchazel Tinctures: These should be combined and applied several times daily to unbroken chilblains, this will help reduce inflammation and heal the skin.

Hypericum, Calendula Tinctures or *Ointment (Hypercal):* Will promote healing of broken chilblains.

Marshmallow, Comfrey Ointments: Will improve the quality of the skin in the area and help to reduce inflammation.

Tamus Mother Tincture (made from *Bryony*): This is useful if applied as soon as the chilblains appear, bringing relief from itching.

HOMOEOPATHY

Constitutional treatment is required to improve the circulation, and the following remedies may offer some specific relief.

Agaricus 6: Is indicated for burning and itching which is aggravated by the cold. Take one twice daily for ten days.

Calc fluor 6X: Improves the elasticity of the blood vessel walls and helps improve the circulation, it is indicated where cracks appear on the surface of the chilblains. One morning and night for ten days.

Ferr Phos 6X: For inflammation and to prevent infection. Three times a day when redness, heat and swelling is present.

Pulsatilla 6: For itching and burning which is worse for warmth. One twice daily for ten days.

AROMATHERAPY

Chamomile, Ginger, Lavender, Lemon: These will reduce inflammation, soothe the pain and itching, promoting cell regeneration. Add a few drops to a vegetable base oil, massage in morning and night, or use a few drops in a foot bath.

CIRCULATION

Circulation is the constant flow of blood and other body fluids in the organism. If there is an imbalance in this flow it can lead to many disorders; including cramp, angina pectoris, high blood pressure, low blood pressure, thrombosis and varicose veins. Poor circulation is particularly associated with heart problems, degeneration of the blood vessels and increased blood viscosity. It is most notably true of circulatory disease that prevention is better than trying to cure a worn out body that is manifesting symptoms. To prevent any circulatory diseases, lifestyle should be considered.

Diet is crucial; there should be a low intake of animal fats, meat, butter, oils, cakes and dairy products. Salt should be avoided, and increase foods rich in vitamin C. Regular, although not necessarily strenuous, exercise is important to tone the circulation. It is also advisable to stop smoking and keep the intake of alcohol to a moderate amount.

There is a close correlation between the levels of stress in life, and problems occurring in the cardio-vascular system. Therefore it is necessary to deal with the underlying causes of stress and tension as well as its physical manifestation. There are many forms of relaxation and emotional integration therapies available at the present time and these may be of great benefit when trying to improve physical and psychological health. Sudden changes in previously established circulation patterns should be assessed by a physician. Acupuncture is particularly recommended for this complaint.

HERBS

For circulatory problems it is advisable to consult a practitioner.

Buckwheat Tea: Will help strengthen the blood vessels and should be drunk on a regular basis. Similarly, *Rutin* tablets could be a useful support.

Dandelion Leaves, Motherwort: If the heart is weak and fails to circulate blood efficiently through the kidneys, or when the blood vessels are weak; a build up of water in certain areas of the body may occur. Combine and drink three times a day for one month.

Hawthorn Berries, Hawthorn Tops: These make a useful heart tonic, drink an infusion three times daily for six weeks.

Horse Chestnut: This is a useful circulatory stimulant, and may be added to the above mixture, when the peripheral circulation is in need of stimulation.

HOMOEOPATHY

Again most benefit will be gained by constitutional treatment from a practitioner. In cases where support for another therapy is required, the following remedies may prove useful:

Calc Fluor 6X: Will strengthen and give elasticity to the blood vessel walls. Take one three times daily for two weeks.

Calc Phos 6X: For those who are generally run down, with slow and weak circulation. Two a day for two weeks.

China, Cactus, Crataegus Tincture: A circulation tonic. Put five drops in water and take three times a day for two months.

Kali Mur 6X: For sluggish circulation and tendency of blood to clot too quickly. One twice daily for two weeks.

AROMATHERAPY

Lavender, Marjoram, Ylang Ylang: Useful oils for high blood pressure, being soothing and calming. They will help to relieve tension and promote relaxation.

Cypress, Ginger, Grapefruit: These are good general circulation tonifiers. Add two to three drops of the essential oils to a warm bath or dilute in a vegetable oil base and massage into the skin.

COLDS

Colds are an attempt by the body to express disharmony. They are an opportunity for the system to discharge unwanted waste matter. They may also be an indication that the person needs to slow down and rest, or to look at some unexpressed emotional difficulties; colds after all share many of the symptoms of grief, e.g. weeping. Thus the aim of treatment should not be to suppress the indicator (and stay out of balance), but to gently restore health and harmony.

Because many of the symptoms of a cold are due to increased mucous secretion, attention to diet is advisable. In particular eliminating all dairy products, wheat products, and concentrated orange juice. It will also help to increase intake of foods that are natural sources of vitamin C, i.e. fresh fruit and vegetables. Unnaturally high doses of vitamin C appear to suppress cold symptoms without allowing the body to continue its elimination processes.

HERBS

Elderflower, Peppermint, Yarrow: This useful mixture combines decongestant, diaphoretic and stimulating properties. Make an infusion and drink a cupful three times a day. If feverishness is marked, add *Boneset.* Add *Red Sage* if there is throat inflammation. Hot *Lemon* and *Honey* is also recommended. Freshly grated *Ginger* may be added to any of the above infusions for a warming effect.

HOMOEOPATHY

ABC 6 (Aconite, Belladonna, Chamomilla): A combination remedy. For the beginning of colds and feverish types of illnesses. Will keep you going during the first stages of a cold, and may prevent it from dragging on too long. Take three times a day for two to three days.

Aconite 6: Sudden onset of cold symptoms, after exposure to cold or cold winds. Sneezing, headache, sore throat and restlessness may be present. One three times a day for two to three days.

Kali Mur 6X: If there is white mucous and general congested feeling. One three times a day for three to four days.

Nat Mur 6X: Watery nasal discharge, also eyes may water. Loss of taste and smell. One three times a day for three to four days.

AROMATHERAPY

Basil, Eucalyptus, Peppermint, Pine, Rosemary: Choose one or two from these essential oils, add to a vegetable base oil, and massage onto the chest. A few drops may be put onto a handkerchief or pillow, or alternatively added to hot water as a steam inhalation.

Ginger: Add ten drops to a basin of warm water for a footbath.

COLD SORES

Many people suffer from this virus, which does not manifest itself until the resistance of the body is lowered, and results in blisters forming around the mouth, or occasionally nose and eyes. The blisters start as reddish lumps and develop into watery vesicles before a scab forms. Constitutional treatment is recommended to deal with the underlying cause, although the following may relieve the occasional sore.

HERBS

Internal

Cleavers, Echinacea, Poke Root: A decoction of equal parts taken twice a day.

External

Golden Seal, Myrrh Tincture: These dabbed on the sores will speed healing.

Calendula Tincture (Hypercal), Hypericum: These are soothing and healing.

Comfrey Ointment: This will help the skin after the scabs have gone.

HOMOEOPATHY

Ars Alb 6: Sores are accompanied by a burning sensation, and sense of irritability. One twice daily for five to ten days.

Hepar Sulph 6: Sores with pus formation, acutely sensitive to touch and cold. One twice daily for five to ten days.

Nat Mur 6X: Herpes blisters containing clear liquid, lips may be cracked, sores often appear during a cold. Take one three times daily for three to four days.

Rhus Tox 6: Inflamed blisters filled with yellowish, watery fluid; associated with burning and itching. One twice daily for five days.

AROMATHERAPY

Lavender: Apply undiluted to the affected area.

COLIC

Colic is generally experienced as a spasmodic pain in the abdomen. In a baby it is usually a digestive upset causing the baby to cry in pain and pass wind. Most infants outgrow it in

43

three to four months, but this can be distressing at the time. In older children and adults a warm hot water bottle hugged to the stomach often gives relief. One should consult a practitioner if it is a recurring symptom, or if there is any doubt about the diagnosis.

HERBS

Caraway, Fennel, Ginger, Wild Yam: Make an infusion and drink as often as necessary.

Caraway, Dill Seeds: For babies these can help to relieve the gripe pains. Use one teaspoon, for one third of a pint. Infuse and give to the baby in a bottle or by teaspoon after feeding.

Chamomile: A soothing tea useful for babies and young children. Make an infusion to drink when required.

HOMOEOPATHY

Chamomilla 6: Restless and irritable, due to a pain in the stomach, and may be accompanied by diarrhoea. Take one three times a day or as necessary. Useful for young children.

Colocynth 6: Violent griping pains in stomach and abdomen. Patient bends double to alleviate the pain. Flatulent colic. Repeat as required.

Mag Phos 6X: Helps colic that is better from warmth and gently rubbing the abdomen. Cramping, spasmodic pains. One every few hours as necessary.

AROMATHERAPY

Basil, Chamomile, Peppermint: Blend a few drops of each with almond oil and gently massage into the stomach.

COLITIS

Colitis is an inflammation of part of the colon or large intestine. It is an increasingly common disturbance of our modern high-stress lifestyle. If the problem is longstanding or with a hereditary background, only persistent careful treatment by a qualified therapist will be of lasting benefit. This condition will respond to a change of diet; based upon non-acidic, non-irritant foods. Avoid dairy products, bran products, pulses, rich fatty foods, and stimulants such as tea, coffee and alcohol.

Symptoms are marked by colicky pains after eating, with constipation or diarrhoea and depression. Check with a doctor for an accurate diagnosis for these symptoms are shared by other illnesses. Colitis can respond quickly to alternative methods of treatment.

Acupuncture has been found to be of much benefit. Also any sufferer of colitis could investigate the Bach Flower Remedies® to assist in bringing about change in the stress patterns and mental habits which lie in the background of this problem.

HERBS

The following herbs may bring relief and ease discomfort.

Comfrey Root, Fenugreek, Marigold, Marshmallow Root, Meadow-sweet: Infuse and drink three times a day.

Slippery Elm: A teaspoon dissolved in warm water taken three times a day.

HOMOEOPATHY

Constitutional treatment with a qualified practitioner is recommended for this condition.

AROMATHERAPY

A relaxing massage and advice from an experienced aroma-therapist will be of benefit.

CONCUSSION

A fall or blow to the head resulting in confusion or temporary loss of consciousness; this may cause a severe disturbance in the body and symptoms can be delayed for several hours. This condition is serious and experienced medical help is required immediately.

Arnica 30 or 200, or *Rescue Remedy*® may be helpful to administer whilst help is being sought.

CONJUNCTIVITIS

An inflammation and swelling of the conjunctiva of the eye. The affected eye will water and look bloodshot. When infected by cold viruses the discharge is clear and watery; bacterial infections result in thick, yellow-green discharges; allergic conjunctivitis is accompanied by itching.

When the discharge dries during sleep the eyelids may stick together.

When treating the eyes take care to wash utensils and hands carefully, and use cool, boiled or distilled water only to apply to the area.

If symptoms persist beyond three days, or if they are associated with any loss of vision, or pain in the eye, or following an injury or possible exposure to flying fragments of metal or grit, then seek urgent medical advice.

(See also: EYE INJURIES, EYE STRAIN.)

HERBS

Internal

Cleavers, Echinacea, Eyebright, Golden Seal: Use a combination of these herbs to fight the infection and detoxify the system. Make a decoction by simmering a teaspoon of the mixed herbs to a mug of water for ten minutes. Strain and drink a cupful three times a day for up to two weeks.

External

Chamomile, Elderflowers, Eyebright, Golden Seal, Marigold: Use these herbs singly or in combination. Make an infusion using a heaped teaspoon of herb to a teacup of boiling water and stand until cool. Strain and use the solution to bathe the eye.

HOMOEOPATHY

Apis 6: Swelling and puffiness of the eyelids. Stinging and burning pains in the eye worse in a warm room. Redness. One dose three times a day for three days.

Belladonna 6: Throbbing sensation. Redness, inflammation and hot, watery, discharge. One dose three times a day for three days.

Euphrasia 6: Acrid tears, thick discharge, sensation of sand in the eye. One dose three times a day for three days.

Pulsatilla 6: Thick, yellow-green discharge. Itching and burning sensation. Often following a cold. Symptoms better in the fresh air. One dose three times a day for three days.

External

Euphrasia Tincture: Add three of four drops of the tincture to a little cool, boiled water and bathe the affected eye.

AROMATHERAPY

Chamomile: Add two drops of the essential oil to a little cool, boiled water. Dip in a piece of cotton wool and hold over the affected eye.

CONSTIPATION

There is much controversy as to how often it is 'healthy' or 'normal' to pass a stool. Generally speaking if bowel movements are less frequent than every two days, or straining is required, and stomach pains are evident, then constipation is present to some extent.

We get many people in the shop requiring laxatives. These are unadviseable as they can be habit forming, and inhibit the bowels' normal functioning. There are two main forms of laxative: one irritates the walls of the colon causing expulsion of waste matter, the other absorbs moisture from the intestinal lining thereby increasing fluids in the forming stools.

Constipation can be helped by a change of diet, increasing fluid intake, fresh fruit and vegetables. Exercise is of great help, and it will also be useful to look at any underlying emotional tensions or stress.

An ongoing change in a previously established pattern of bowel habit should be assessed by a physician.

HERBS

Buckthorn, Cascara Sagrada, Fennel, Ginger, Liquorice, Marsh-mallow, Root, Rhubarb Root, Senna Leaves: Make an infusion and drink one cup a day, in the evening. This will alleviate the odd bout of constipation. Anything more persistant should be referred to a herbalist.

HOMOEOPATHY

If this complaint is chronic, seek advice from a trained practitioner. For acute cases the following may be of help.

Alumina 6 or 30: Inactivity of the colon, with soft stool; constipation common to travellers. Take three doses of the 6th potency a day for five days, or one dose of the 30th potency a day for three days.

Nat Mur 6X: Constipation when caused from lack of moisture in the intestines. Hard, dry, black, lumpy stools difficult to pass, accompanied by dull, heavy headache. Take one three times a day for three days.

Nux Vom 6: Urging for stool that does not come. A small stool may be passed, with the feeling some is left behind. One or two doses.

Sepia 6: Ineffectual urging, sensation of lump in the rectum, not relieved by passing a stool. Feeling of heaviness and sluggishness. Constipation of pregnancy. One or two doses.

AROMATHERAPY

There are many essential oils to help tone, detoxify and relax the body. Massage would be of great benefit to relieve tension and a visit to an aromatherapist is recommended.

Fennel, Rosemary: In an acute situation, these oils diluted in a massage base oil and rubbed on the abdomen may help.

BACH FLOWER REMEDIES®

These could be very useful to change habits, and help underlying emotional or stress patterns. See the list in the Appendix or consult a practitioner.

CONVALESCENCE

After a debilitating illness or a long winter when the body's natural defences have been weakened and one is prone to illness and infections, the following may be of help.
(See also: APPETITE LOSS.)

HERBS

Balm, Borage, Nettle, Vervain: These will soothe and gently tonify the system. Combine and make an infusion to drink three times a day.

Slippery Elm: Take if the digestion is weak.

HOMOEOPATHY

Calc Phos 6X: Is of great help as it tones up the system and aids the assimilation processes. Take three times a day for two weeks.

Phos Ac 30: For exhaustion and apathy, following trauma or illness. Take only two doses eight hours apart.

AROMATHERAPY

Geranium, Lavender, Melissa, Rosemary: Choose one or two of these oils and add a couple of drops to a warm bath, or apply diluted in a massage base.

CORNS

These are often formed by pressure from ill-fitting shoes, and poor posture, creating a hard layer of dead tissue, which can be quite painful. It is advisable to visit a chiropodist if the corns are at all severe.

Soak the foot in very hot water until the skin becomes soft, and gently peel away dead tissue.

HERBS

Calendula Tincture, Hypericum: These added to the water promote healing and prevent infection.
Comfrey, Marshmallow, Slippery Elm, Garlic: Infused and applied as a compress may be of help.
Lemon Juice: Also softens the skin.

HOMOEOPATHY

Calc Fluor 6X: For hard, calloused skin. Take twice daily for ten days.
Ferr Phos 6X: For acute inflammatory pain. One three times a day.

AROMATHERAPY

Lavender, Lemon, Marigold (Tagetes): Combine and add a few drops to a warm foot bath. This combination of oils may also be diluted in a vegetable base oil and massaged into the foot.
Tea Tree: Apply undiluted and massage into the corn to relieve pain and prevent infection.

COUGHS

Coughing is a reflex action as an attempt to expel foreign matter from the air passages. Mucous is produced as a response to dust, bacterial infection and other irritants. Arresting a cough by use of cough suppressants is therefore undesirable, and can cause a deeper infection. Avoid dairy products and other mucous-forming foods. A simple and soothing cough remedy can be made from fresh lemon, honey, and a few drops of glycerine dissolved in hot water.
(See also: ASTHMA, BRONCHITIS, WHOOPING COUGH.)

CRAMP

This is a painful spasm of muscles which may be due to circulatory problems. Consult a practitioner if the cramping occurs frequently.
(See also: COLIC, MENSTRUAL DISORDERS.)

HERBS

Balm, Cramp Bark: These herbs as an infusion may help to alleviate the problem. Drink a cupful as required.

HOMOEOPATHY

Arnica 6: Cramp after over-exertion of muscles; system feels sore and bruised. One dose as necessary.
Cuprum 6: Severe cramping of the extremities, worse at night. One dose as required.

Mag Phos 6X: For muscular, stomach and menstrual cramps. Alleviated by rubbing and warmth. Dosage as required.

AROMATHERAPY

Aniseed, Basil, Marjoram: Add two drops of each to a little base massage oil, and rub into the area.

CROUP

A harsh cough accompanied by rapid, loud breathing; occurs mostly in children at night. Emergency care is needed if symptoms have no relief after twenty minutes, or whenever the child has severe breathing difficulties. Be cautious: this is a potentially serious condition. A traditional remedy is to provide a steamy atmosphere by boiling a kettle in the room.

HERBS

Eucalyptus: This may be used as an inhalation. Put some of the leaves in a basin, pour on boiling water, and stand it in the patient's room.

Catnip, Chamomile, Coltsfoot, Marshmallow Leaves: A soothing tea that will also relieve spasms. Make an infusion and drink a cupful as required.

HOMOEOPATHY

Aconite 30: At onset, if there is a lot of fear and worse at midnight. One or two doses as required.

Hepar Sulph 30, Spongia 30: If *Aconite* brings no relief. Child wakes feeling suffocated, with loud violent cough and loss of voice. *Spongia* is worse before midnight and *Hepar Sulph* afterwards. One or two doses as required.

AROMATHERAPY

Cypress, Eucalyptus: These two oils could be diluted and sprayed in the room, or placed in a bowl of hot water to inhale the steam.

Lavender: Can be used as a compress to soothe the child, apply on the head or chest.

BACH FLOWER REMEDIES®

Rescue Remedy®: This may help a fearful child.

CYSTITIS

A urinary tract infection which can be most uncomfortable. The symptoms are an urgent need to urinate, frequency of urination, accompanied by burning sensation. If there is fever, lower back pain, blood or sediment in the urine, we advise you to seek medical attention, as the kidneys may be infected, leading to chronic damage.

Professional help should be sought if the condition is recurrent. The following remedies may help a mild, acute attack. Barley water made from pot (not pearl) barley, drunk frequently should help, as should taking salt baths.

HERBS

Buchu, Cornsilk, Couchgrass, Marshmallow Leaves: Combine, infuse and drink a cupful every two hours.

HOMOEOPATHY

Apis 30: Frequent urge to urinate, last few drops sting. Two or three doses.

Cantharis 30: Persistant and violent urge to urinate, with burning, cutting or stabbing pains. Two or three doses.

Merc Cor 6: Urine is a dark colour, burning sensation. Worse at night. Two or three doses for three days.

Nux Vom 6 or 30: Cutting, burning pains; feels chilly and irritable. Worse at night. Take three doses of the 6th potency a day for five days, or one dose of the 30th potency a day for three days.

AROMATHERAPY

Bergamot, Cedarwood, Cypress, Juniper, Sandalwood: Combine two drops of *Sandalwood* with one each of the other oils in a little of a massage base oil and apply to the abdomen to relieve the discomfort.

Lavender: Add ten drops to a warm bath. This will be soothing and help fight the infection.

Wind Flower
(Anemone Pulsatilla)

DANDRUFF

Dandruff seems to be an indication of your general state of health. It is in fact dead cells flaking from the scalp. Strong detergents as in anti-dandruff shampoos should be avoided as they are only a short-term solution and may cause scalp irritation if used frequently. Mild shampoos such as *Nettle* are recommended. Best results will come from a visit to a qualified practitioner especially when dandruff is severe.

HERBS

External

Nettles: Make an infusion and massage into scalp daily.

Internal

Burdock, Heartsease: Mix and make an infusion using one teaspoon per cup. Drink three cups a day.

HOMOEOPATHY

Homoeopathic tissue salts may be helpful.
Kali Mur 6X: Copious white dandruff. One dose morning and night for ten days.

Kali Sulph 6X: Poor conditions of scalp with flaking and scaling. Yellow dandruff. One dose morning and night for ten days.

AROMATHERAPY

Cedarwood, Lavender, Rosemary: Add ten drops of each to a suitable vegetable base oil, e.g. coconut oil. Massage into scalp, leave on overnight before washing off. Will help improve the condition of hair and scalp.

DENTAL PROBLEMS

(See also: ABSCESS, GUM PROBLEMS, TEETHING, TOOTH-ACHE.)

HOMOEOPATHY

Arnica 30: This remedy can considerably lessen the physical trauma and aid recovery following a visit to the dentist. Take one dose one hour before treatment and one dose one hour afterwards.

BACH FLOWER REMEDIES®

Mimulus: For anticipatory fear. Take a couple of drops in a little water as often as required before visiting the dentist.

DEPRESSION

There are many interpretations of what depression means. We recognise that there are times when states of feeling low and unhappy with yourself and the world hit you unsuspectingly.

Some physical reasons can provoke this state; such as after giving birth, after illness, after an operation or as a result of taking drugs, etc. We will list some helpful remedies to take when there is an obvious cause, or when the depression is of a non-severe nature; but basically we feel that much depression springs from an attitude that is common in our society in which we tend to lose touch with our purpose for existence and our inner sense of creativity. We will use difficult circumstances and various incidents as the excuse, but really we feel that depression is the outcome of lack of communication of initial emotional reactions. Failure or inability to recognise and express these primary emotions leads to suppression; this develops into a complication and confusion of emotions, which may progress into feelings of depression and a loss of our sense of worth.

Some symptoms of depression are; loss of appetite, sleeplessness, anxiety, lassitude and lack of sexual interest.

The use of anti-depressants we feel is counter productive. There are nowadays many forms of group or individual therapy which may be of help. Some assessment should be made (by a qualified practitioner) of the severity of the depression: in particular regarding the presence of suicidal ideas. Milder forms of depression can usually be treated by a combination of psychotherapy and other approaches, but more severe depression may need more intensive intervention, possibly including twenty-four hour care under professional supervision.

HERBS

Balm, Scullcap, St John's Wort, Vervain, Wild Oat: These herbs are useful and soothing nervines. Mix the herbs and make an infusion using one heaped teaspoonful of herbs to a cupful of boiling water. This may be drunk three times a day.

Kola: Add this to the above mixture if there is weakness and debility associated with the depression.

Best results will be obtained from a visit to a qualified herbalist.

HOMOEOPATHY

We feel that when dealing with depression, any homoeopathic remedy should be prescribed by a qualified homoeopath, as it is constitutional treatment that will be of lasting benefit.

AROMATHERAPY

A course of treatment by a qualified aromatherapist could be of great value in cases of depression.

Basil, Clary Sage, Jasmine, Neroli, Rose: These oils have an uplifting effect. Add a few drops of the one of your choice to an essential oil burner and fragrance the room, or add a couple of drops to a warm bath.

BACH FLOWER REMEDIES®

Bach Flower Remedies® can be of great benefit in the treatment of depression. We suggest that you spend some time going through the relevant literature and choosing the appropriate remedies for yourself. Alternatively, one may visit a practitioner for guidance about the most useful remedies to take.

DIARRHOEA

There are many causes of diarrhoea. Chronic (long-term) diarrhoea as experienced for example in colitis or diverticulitis should be referred to a qualified practitioner. Unfamiliar or spoilt foods can cause an inflammation or irritation of the stomach lining or intestinal tract; diarrhoea will result as an attempt to eliminate them. Emotional circumstances such as grief, exam tension etc. or travelling may also cause diarrhoea.

If the diarrhoea is severe, or if it continues for more than twenty-four hours, consult a medical practitioner because diarrhoea can be an indication of something more serious. It is extremely important to alert a medical practitioner about any case of diarrhoea occurring in babies and young children, as dehydration can set in quickly, and this is a very dangerous situation: if in doubt this is a time when it is vital to err on the side of caution.

General care includes drinking plenty of water and eating only plain foods until the digestive system has had a chance to settle down.

HERBS

Chamomile, Marshmallow, Meadowsweet: Combine the above herbs and make an infusion using one heaped teaspoon of herbs to a cupful of boiling water. Drink a cupful every few hours to soothe irritation and counteract any acidity.

Ginger, Peppermint: Add these to any of the above if griping pains are present.

Sage: An infusion may be drunk after a light meal to aid digestion and reduce diarrhoea.

Slippery Elm: Stir a heaped teaspoonful of Slippery Elm powder into a cup of warm water. Drink a cupful three times a day. This will soothe the digestive system and provide some nourishment.

HOMOEOPATHY

There are many homoeopathic remedies for diarrhoea and if you are registered with a homoeopathic practitioner it is best to consult them for advice, this is a must when dealing with young children. The following remedies are some of those most commonly found to be of assistance in treating diarrhoea. For best results it may be necessary to try two or three different remedies as the symptoms change.

Ars Alb 30: Watery, burning diarrhoea. Results of bad food or excessive eating of fruit. The patient is restless, anxious and chilly, and desires sips of water. One dose every few hours as required.

Bryonia 30: Gushing diarrhoea worse whenever the patient moves. Dry parched lips and great thirst. Take two or three doses spread throughout the day.

Chamomilla 6 or 30: Diarrhoea in children. Colicky pains, green or watery stool. The child is whiney and irritable.

59

Colocynth 30: Diarrhoea resulting from food poisoning with cramping, colicky pains. The pains are better for pressure and bending double. One dose every few hours as required.

Mag Phos 30: Cramping pains accompanying diarrhoea. The patient is chilly. One dose every few hours as required.

Merc Sol 30: Offensive, smelly, watery, bloody or mucousy stools. Constant urging and straining to pass a stool. Diarrhoea worse at night. Two or three doses spread over one or two days.

Nat Phos 30: Sour-smelling, acidic stools. Summer diarrhoea from eating too much fruit. One dose every few hours as required.

Podophyllum 30: Gushing, watery stools passed painlessly. Gurgling in the abdomen. Diarrhoea worse after eating or drinking, and worse in hot weather. One dose every few hours as required.

Pulsatilla 30: Diarrhoea after rich food. Patient dislikes a stuffy room and is worse at night. Thirstless, depressed and weepy patient. One dose every few hours as required.

AROMATHERAPY

Chamomile, Geranium, Sandalwood: Add a few drops of any of these oils to a vegetable oil base and lightly massage onto the abdomen to soothe the digestive tract.

Thyme: This oil may be sprayed in the room as a disinfectant.

E

Purple Cone Flower
(Echinacea)

EARACHE

Earache is particularly common in children, it is often a painful and distressing problem. Pain is caused by inflammation, or a build up of fluids causing pressure on the eardrum. Infection of the middle ear, which is indicated by redness and swelling in the outer ear, can be serious and we suggest you get medical attention as soon as possible. Any pain or swelling in the bony area behind or under the ear requires immediate medical attention as this may develop into inflammation of the brain which is an extremely dangerous condition. The presence of a discharge from the ear indicates a perforation of the ear drum. Care must be taken to prevent the entry of water, shampoo, etc., until the drum has fully healed.

Any residual hearing loss, after the acute episode is over, should be professionally assessed: this can easily go unnoticed in children. Recurrent earaches can result in permanent hearing loss so constitutional treatment by a qualified alternative therapist should be considered to prevent attacks recurring.

HERBS

Chamomile, Echinacea, Golden Rod, Golden Seal: Combine the herbs and make a decoction using one teaspoon of herbs to a cupful of water and simmer for ten minutes. Drink a cupful three times a day to reduce inflammation and prevent infection. Children may not like this bitter mixture so it may be worth using herbal tinctures instead: combine the tinctures and dilute a teaspoon of the tincture in a wine glass of warm water to drink three times a day.

Garlic Oil, Mullein Oil: Add a few drops slightly warmed to a piece of cotton wool and place gently inside the outer ear.

HOMOEOPATHY

Aconite 6 or 30: Sudden attack of earache after exposure to cold winds. One 6 potency every few hours for two to three days, or two doses of the 30 potency eight hours apart.

Belladonna 6 or 30: Throbbing pain in the ear. Ear looks red and feels hot. Pain accompanied with fever. Dosage as for *Aconite.*

Chamomilla 6 or 30: Earache in teething children. Child is whiney and intolerant, the pain feels unbearable to them. One cheek looks red. Dosage as for *Aconite.*

Ferrum Phos 6X: Helpful at the beginning stage of inflammation when there are few distinguishing features. Ear feels hot and looks red. One dose every three hours.

Hepar Sulph 6 or 30: Useful when pus has formed. Stitching pains in the ear. Pains are worse at night. Patient is feverish, irritable and sweaty. Dosage as for *Aconite.*

Kali Mur 6X or 30: Blocked up feeling in the ear; diminished hearing. This may be useful after the pain has subsided but hearing is impaired. One dose of 6X potency three times a day for five days or just two doses of 30 potency eight hours apart.

Pulsatilla 6 or 30: Pain as from pressure in the ear. Pains worse from warmth and at night. Child is weepy and craves attention. Thick yellow discharge. Dosage as for *Aconite.*

Silica 6 or 30: Pain and swelling in the area around the ear.

Yellow or green discharge. Weak, tired and chilly patient. Dosage as for *Aconite*.

AROMATHERAPY

Lavender: Put two or three drops on a piece of cotton wool and hold against the ear to soothe pain and reduce inflammation. Or dilute *Lavender Oil* in a massage base to gently massage in around the ear area.

ECZEMA

Eczema is a name given to a wide variety of skin disorders. As it is a deep-rooted condition with a variety of causes, it should be treated constitutionally by a qualified practitioner. Herbalism, naturopathy, homoeopathy and aromatherapy can all be very successful in dealing with this distressing problem. Symptoms include redness, itching, flaking and weeping skin. The use of strong chemical ointments, whilst effective in the short term, have serious long term side-effects and are not curative, merely suppressive.

The following suggestions may be used in conjunction with remedies prescribed by a qualified practitioner, but check with them first.

HERBS

Internal

Burdock, Chamomile, Chickweed, Heartsease, Fumitory, Marigold, Red Clover: Combine the above herbs, make an infusion using one teaspoon of herbs to one teacupful of boiling water, and drink a cupful three times a day for up to six weeks.
Borage, Echinacea, Wild Yam: These may be added to help strengthen the immune system.

External

Chickweed, Marigold: Make an infusion using one tablespoon of herbs to one pint of boiling water. Leave to stand until cool, strain, then bathe the affected areas.

Calendula Ointment: A soothing and healing ointment that will help prevent infection.

Stellaria Ointment: This will help soothe any itching.

HOMOEOPATHY

We recommend that you see a qualified homoeopath to get the full benefit of homoeopathic treatment.

AROMATHERAPY

Chamomile, Geranium, Lavender: Combine the oils. Use as a compress, in a warm bath, or dilute in a suitable vegetable massage oil to apply to the affected parts.

EYE INJURIES

Because the eyes are so delicate, any eye injury should be examined by a physician for possible complications. Loose foreign bodies in the eye should be flushed out with plenty of cool, clean water.

(See also: CONJUNCTIVITIS.)

HERBS

Witchazel: Dilute distilled *Witchazel* in cool, boiled water. Dip some clean cotton wool in the solution and hold over the eye to soothe inflammation and bruising.

Chamomile, Eyebright: An infusion may be drunk to strengthen the eyes and reduce inflammation.

Tinctures

Euphrasia: Use to soothe irritation or inflammation. Add three to four drops of the tincture to a little cool, boiled water in an eyebath and gently bathe the eyes.

Calendula (Hypercal), Hypericum: Use after a foreign body has been expelled to soothe the eye and help prevent infection. Add three or four drops to a little cool, boiled water and use as an eyewash.

HOMOEOPATHY

Arnica 6 or 30: Useful following any injury. Prevents haemorrhage, reduces bruising and helps with shock.

Ledum 30: For a black eye with bruising and swelling. Take two or three doses over two days.

Silica 6X: Will help to expel a foreign body from the eye. One dose three times a day.

Symphytum 6 or 30: For injury to the eyeball. One dose of 30 potency a day for three days, or three doses of 6 potency a day for five days.

AROMATHERAPY

Chamomile, Lavender: Add one drop of each oil to an eyebath with cool, boiled water in. Dip in a piece of cotton wool and hold over the affected eye.

EYE STRAIN

Cold teabags, placed on the eye are very effective.

HERBS

Chamomile: Make an infusion and cool. Strain and bathe the eye if sore or inflamed.

Eyebright: Make an infusion, cool, strain and bathe the eye. This tea can also be taken internally to strengthen the eyes.

Tinctures

Euphrasia: Add three or four drops of the tincture to a little cool, boiled water in an eyebath and gently bathe the eyes.

HOMOEOPATHY

Ruta 6: Eyes red, hot and painful from reading fine print, sewing, etc. Vision seems dim. One dose three times a day for five days.

AROMATHERAPY

Chamomile, Lavender: Two drops of each used as a compress, cool or warm. If swelling is present use a cold compress.

F

Deadly Nightshade ~ (Atropa belladonna)

FAINTING

This is a reflex action as a result of temporary loss of oxygen to the brain; often resulting from intense fear, low blood pressure, lack of air, e.g., stuffy room, emotional upset, or intense pain. Basic first-aid can be given: Sit with head lower than body until one feels better. If fainting recurs, seek medical advice.

HERBS

Peppermint, Rosemary, St John's Wort: Any of these can be used as a tea for occasional fainting. Make an infusion and drink a cupful every two to three hours.

HOMOEOPATHY

Chamomilla 6 or 30: Fainting from severe pain. Use one or more doses as required.
Chinchona 6 or 30: Fainting due to loss of blood. Use one or more dose as required.
Coffea 6 or 30: Fainting from excitement. Use one or more doses as required.
Ignatia 6 or 30: Fainting due to emotional shock or hysteria. Use one or more doses as required.

Pulsatilla 6 or 30: Fainting from hot, stuffy atmosphere. Use one or more doses as required.

AROMATHERAPY

Peppermint, Rosemary: Either of these can be used placed on a pad of cotton wool and held under the nose.

BACH FLOWER REMEDIES®

Rescue Remedy®: Take a few drops as required.

FEVER

This is a natural defence of the body to combat disease, marked by an increase in body temperature. As long as the temperature does not rise too high it is best to let the fever run its course, as this will allow the body to heal itself. For a mild fever the following remedies will assist; remembering plenty of fluids should be taken and chilliness prevented. Sponging the body with tepid water will help. If fever continues to rise, consult a physician.

It is especially important to keep a close watch on children, as they may develop convulsions during a high fever and emergency medical advice must be sought if there seems any likelihood of this occurring.

HERBS

Boneset, Echinacea, Elderflower, Yarrow: Combine and drink an infusion three times a day to reduce fever and help fight off infection.

Balm, Chamomile: This can also be drunk as a soothing tea throughout a fever.

HOMOEOPATHY

Aconite 30: For sudden onset after exposure to cold wind. Anxious, fearful, dry skin and mouth. Take one dose of the 30th potency and repeat if necessary.

Ars Alb 6 or 30: Fluctuating temperature, restless, anxious, fearful, chilly patient. Thirsty for sips of water. Take three doses of the 6th potency a day for five days, or one dose of the 30th potency a day for three days.

Belladonna 30: Restless, agitated, glassy eyes, red face, burning hot skin and delirium. Take one dose of the 30th potency and repeat if necessary.

Ferrum Phos 30: Fever accompanied by throbbing head. Take one dose of the 30th potency a day for three days.

Gelsemum 30: Drowsy, aching, chilly, heavy, no thirst. Take one dose of the 30th potency a day for three days.

Merc Sol 6 or 30: Sweating, worse at night, offensive smell in room, thirsty. Take one dose of the 30th potency a day for three days.

Pulsatilla 30: Fevers in children. Changeable moods, thirstless, desires fresh air. Take one dose of the 30th potency a day for three days.

AROMATHERAPY

Chamomile: Add a few drops to the bath or sponge the patient down from a bowl of water with two to three drops of *Chamomile* added.

Eucalyptus: Add a few drops of water and spray around the room to disinfect it.

FLATULENCE

Gas in the stomach and intestines caused by the intake of air during eating or drinking, or undigested food fermenting; often accompanied by a bloated feeling, abdominal pain, belching and passing gas.

Avoid foods that you know cause this feeling, also don't eat or drink when you are overtired, anxious or angry. Eat slowly, chewing each mouthful well before swallowing.

HERBS

Aniseed, Caraway, Fennel, Peppermint: Any of the above may be taken on their own, or combined and made into an infusion using one teaspoon per cup. Leave to stand for ten minutes, strain and drink after meals.

HOMOEOPATHY

Carbo Veg 6: One dose for repeated belching, bloated sensation in abdomen, belching alleviates the discomfort. Useful in elderly people.
China 6: One dose when stomach feels full of gas, distention, passing wind does not ameliorate.
Lycopodium 6: One dose with fullness even after light eating; rumbling and gurgling in abdomen.
Mag Phos 6: One dose when required for flatulence with much belching of gas and crampy pains.

AROMATHERAPY

Aniseed, Coriander, Fennel, Peppermint: Any of the above oils will help relieve flatulence. Two to three drops diluted in a light vegetable oil base and lightly massaged over the abdomen.

FLU

(See: INFLUENZA.)

FRACTURES

It is often difficult to tell if a bone is broken — an X-ray will be needed, and the bone set rigid in plaster to allow it to heal. The most common sites of fractures are the wrist, ankle and the collar bone. Old people are more prone to fractures if their bones are weakened. The following remedies will promote healing of the bones.

(See also: ACCIDENTS.)

HERBS

Comfrey, Horsetail, Mousear: These herbs are reputed to be able to help the bones to heal faster. Make an infusion using the leaves and apply locally if possible.

Comfrey Root: A decoction of this herb can be taken internally using one teaspoon per cup. Simmer for ten minutes, strain and drink three cups per day, until the bone is healed.

Comfrey Ointment: This may be applied externally.

HOMOEOPATHY

Arnica 200: One dose for shock with bruising, swelling and tenderness.

Eupatorium Perf 6: For aching pain in bones. One dose two times a day for two or three weeks.

Hypericum 200: One dose for agonizing pain involving nerves.

Symphytum 6: Twice daily promotes healing and union of bones. Take for three or four weeks.

AROMATHERAPY

Lavender, Rosemary, Thyme: Combine up to ten drops of each in a 90 ml bottle of a vegetable base oil and gently massage morning and night to help with the aching.

BACH FLOWER REMEDIES®

Rescue Remedy®: This may be given for any shock involved.

FUNGAL INFECTION

(See: ATHLETE'S FOOT, THRUSH.)

G

Couch Grass
(*Agropyron repens*)

GASTRITIS

An inflammation of the lining of the stomach, often caused by poor diet, irritants like tobacco and alcohol, and hurried meals. A stressful lifestyle could also be a major contributory factor.

The symptoms are heartburn, acidic risings and pain in the abdomen. Only easily digested foods should be eaten. It may be useful to visit a naturopath for dietary advice.

HERBS

Comfrey, Marshmallow Leaves, Meadowsweet: Combine in equal parts and make an infusion using one teaspoon of herbs to a cupful of boiling water. Drink three cups a day.

Slippery Elm: A light and soothing nutritional food. Stir a teaspoon of the powdered herb into a little warm water to make a paste, top up the cup with warm water, and drink after each meal, or three times a day.

HOMOEOPATHY

Kali Mur 6X: Indigestion from fatty or rich food. Nausea. Stomach feels heavy. Ameliorated by a cold drink. One dose every few hours when required.

Nat Carb 6: Weak digestion, aggravated by slight errors in the

73

diet. Acidity and belching. Heartburn after fatty food. One dose every few hours as necessary.

Nat Phos 6X: Ailments from excess acidity. Sour eructations. One dose every few hours as required.

Nux Vom 6: Waterbrash, nausea and sour eructations. Pain in the stomach, back and chest. Aggravated by rich food, stimulants and alcohol. One dose every two to three hours as necessary.

Pulsatilla 6: Aggravated by fat and rich food. Nausea and heartburn with a bad taste in the mouth. Thirstlessness. Stomach feels deranged and heavy. One dose every few hours as necessary.

AROMATHERAPY

Aniseed, Basil, Chamomile: Choose one of the above oils. Add a few drops to a little vegetable oil and massage over the abdomen, or add two or three drops of one of the oils to a warm bath.

GASTROENTERITIS

Inflammation of stomach and intestines, which produces symptoms such as abdominal pain, vomiting and diarrhoea. This results from a variety of causes, such as viral, e.g. gastric 'flu, food or metal poisoning and infections. Care must be taken that the person does not become dehydrated and that the normal electrolyte balance of the body is maintained. In a young child failure to hold down clear fluids, drowsiness, disinterest in fluids and decreased passage of urine are all warning signs of the need for urgent professional advice.

Following the first symptoms of gastroenteritis the stomach should be rested for the first eight hours with sips of water being taken; after the first eight hours, to prevent dehydration, plenty of fluids should be taken, possibly with a pinch of salt and sugar added. After twenty-four hours plain, light food may be introduced. If symptoms are not relieved by the following remedies after twenty-four hours, or before that time in young children, seek immediate medical aid.

(See also: DIARRHOEA.)

HERBS

Comfrey Root, Marshmallow Root, Meadowsweet: Make a decoction using a heaped teaspoon of the combined herbs to a cupful of water and simmer for ten minutes. Drink a cupful three times a day.

Slippery Elm: A light and soothing nutritious food. Stir a teaspoon of the herb into a little warm water to make a paste, top up the cup with warm water, and drink three times a day.

HOMOEOPATHY

Ars Alb 6 or 30: Violent vomiting and diarrhoea accompanied with abdominal pains. Chilly, restless, exhausted, fearful and feverish. Burning sensations. Aggravated at night and by eating. Four doses of 6 potency a day for five days or two doses of 30 potency a day for three days.

Belladonna 6 or 30: Acute violent throbbing pains in the stomach accompanied with fever. Dosage as for *Ars Arb.*

Bryonia 6 or 30: Nausea with vomiting and abdominal pain. Pain worse when moving and in the morning. Feels irritable. Better when lying on the stomach. Thirsty with dry mouth. Dosage as for *Ars Alb.*

Colocynth 6 or 30: Severe abdominal pains with vomiting and diarrhoea. Doubles up with the pain and holds the stomach because pressure and warmth bring relief. Feels better after a stool. Dosage as for *Ars Alb.*

Ipecac 6 or 30: Persistant nausea with vomiting, the nausea continues even after vomiting. Patient has a clean tongue. Vomit and stool contains mucous. Dosage as for *Ars Alb.*

Mag Phos 6X or 30: Crampy abdominal pains ameliorated by pressure and warmth. Dosage as for *Ars Alb.*

Nux Vom 6 or 30: Vomiting and retching. Back aches. Chilly, irritable patient. Patient much relieved after vomiting. Dosage as for *Ars Alb.*

75

Phosphorus 6 or 30: Burning pain in the stomach with vomiting. Thirst for cold drinks that are vomited soon after swallowing. Better after sleep. Dosage as for *Ars Alb*.

Podophyllum 6 or 30: Profuse, smelly diarrhoea. Dosage as for *Ars Alb*.

Pulsatilla 6 or 30: Nausea and diarrhoea. Worse at night, and worse in a warm room. Thirstless, craves open air. Children become clingy and weepy. Dosage as for *Ars Alb*.

Veratrum Alb 6 or 30: Cramping pains in the abdomen followed by profuse diarrhoea. Patient covered in cold sweat. Craves cold water and refreshing things which aggravate. Dosage as for *Ars Alb*.

AROMATHERAPY

Chamomile: Add a few drops to a vegetable oil base and lightly massage onto the abdomen.

Thyme: This oil may be sprayed in the room as a disinfectant.

GINGIVITIS

An infection of the surface tissues of the gums, found in association with certain bacteria, which an increase in oral hygiene will help eliminate. Eating refined foods and sugar are contributory causes. This condition must not be neglected as it can lead to weakening of the gums and eventual loss of teeth.

HERBS

Echinacea, Myrrh: Combine and use one teaspoon of each herb; simmer for ten minutes. Strain and allow to cool; use as a mouthwash. The above may be used in tincture form; dilute five drops of each in a glass of warm water and use as a mouthwash.

HOMOEOPATHY

Calendula Tincture: Dilute three drops in warm water and use as a mouthwash.

AROMATHERAPY

Lavender, Myrrh: Add three drops of each to warm boiled water. Use as a mouthwash at least twice a day.

GOUT

A build-up of uric acid around one or two joints, most commonly the big toe, that become swollen and excruciatingly painful.

Diet will be of great importance in the treatment of gout: avoid rich, fatty foods; stimulants including spices, tobacco and alcohol. This condition does have an hereditary factor.

A qualified practitioner should be consulted, and the following remedies may be used as an adjunct to their treatment, with their approval. As well as the three therapies of herbalism, homoeopathy, and aromatherapy, we particularly recommend acupuncture and naturopathy for the treatment of gout.

HERBS

Burdock, Celery Seed, Couchgrass, Dandelion Leaves, Sarsaparilla, Yarrow: Combine the herbs in equal parts. Make an infusion using one teaspoon of herbs to a cupful of boiling water, stand for ten minutes, strain, and drink a cupful three times a day for up to six weeks.

HOMOEOPATHY

Nat Phos 6X, Nat Sulph 6X: These tissue salts will encourage the body to eliminate acid deposits more effectively. Take one of each morning and evening for ten days.

AROMATHERAPY

Benzoin, Juniper, Rosemary: Regular massage with a combination
of these oils will help with the pain and encourage
elimination of the acid deposits. Add a few drops of each to
a light vegetable oil base and gently massage the area
surrounding the painful joint, or add a drop of each to a
little warm water and bathe the area.

H

Hyssop
(Hyssopus officinalis)

HAEMORRHOIDS

Haemorrhoids (or piles) are distended veins in the rectal area, often painless, but they may rupture, bleed, itch or cause pain. Frequent causes are constipation, liver congestion and pregnancy. There is also a hereditary factor. This is a common complaint that can be helped considerably by correct treatment. However, other more serious forms of rectal bleeding may mimic or co-exist with haemorrhoids, consult a physician for a diagnosis.

If constipation is a causative factor, then a naturopath should be consulted for advice on diet. *Rutin* tablets may be added to the diet (or eat more buckwheat) as this will strengthen the capilliary walls.

(See also: VARICOSE VEINS.)

HERBS

Dandelion Root, Golden Seal, Stone Root, Yarrow: Make an infusion using a heaped teaspoon to a cup of boiling water and stand for ten minutes before straining. Drink a cupful three times a day.

Pilewort: An ointment may be made from this herb to apply externally.

Witchazel: Distilled *Witchazel* may be diluted in water and applied externally to soothe inflammation and relieve itching.

HOMOEOPATHY

Arnica 6 or 30: Painful haemorrhoids caused by childbirth or over-straining. Bruised sensation. One 30 a day for three days, or one 6 three times a day for five days.

Calc Fluor 6X: Tendency to lax fibres, varicose veins and piles. Will tone up the elastic tissues. One dose morning and night for ten days.

Collinsonia 6 or 30: Sensation of sharp sticks in the rectum. Painful, bleeding and protruding piles with constipation. One 30 potency a day for three days, or one 6 three times a day for five days.

Hamamelis 6 or 30: Piles, bleeding profusely, with soreness and a bruised feeling. Tendency to varicose veins and piles. one 30 potency a day for three days, or one 6 three times a day for five days.

Nit Ac 6 or 30: Painful, easily bleeding piles. Prolonged pain after stools. Rectum feels torn. One 30 a day for three days or one 6 potency three times a day for five days.

Nux Vomica 6 or 30: Itching piles. Alleviated by cool bathing. Patient is irritable with the pain. One 30 potency a day for three days or one 6 three times a day for five days.

Sulphur 6 or 30: Large haemorrhoids that are sore, tender, raw, burn, bleed and smart. One 30 a day for three days or one 6 three times a day for five days.

AROMATHERAPY

Cypress, Lavender, Myrrh: Add a few drops of any of the above to a warm bath or apply as a local compress.

HANGOVERS

An over-indulgence in alcohol puts a great strain on the liver, which attempts to process all the toxins. As so many alcoholic drinks these days are laced with dubious chemicals this will put an added strain on the liver. Obviously people with a weakness in this organ would be well advised to avoid all alcohol.

Symptoms of a hangover include headache, dry mouth, thirst, irritability and nausea. The following remedies will offer relief for an occasional hangover; if these complaints occur regularly then counselling regarding alcoholism tendencies should be considered.

HERBS

Balm, Chamomile, Dandelion Leaves, Meadowsweet, Yarrow: A combination of these herbs will encourage the body to eliminate toxins and be soothing for any headache or nausea. Make an infusion using a heaped teaspoon of the mixed herbs to a cupful of boiling water. Drink a cupful every few hours.

HOMOEOPATHY

Cocculus 6: Dizziness and nausea, drowsiness. Especially after excessive drinking of beer. One dose every few hours.
Nat Phos 6X: Will relieve symptoms of dehydration. Counteracts acidity (after excessive drinking of wine). One dose every few hours.
Nat Sulph 6X: Assists the liver in eliminating toxins. Dull heavy headache. One dose every few hours.
Nux Vom 6: Oversensitivity to noise. Irritability, nausea. General effects of over-indulgence of food, alcohol, tobacco or stimulants. One dose every few hours.

AROMATHERAPY

Basil, Grapefruit, Juniper, Rosemary: Add one drop of each to a warm bath, or add a couple of drops of each to a little vegetable base oil for a massage.

HAYFEVER

Hayfever is a common complaint, usually a seasonal allergy caused by higher levels of pollen in the air. The usual symptoms which include sneezing, runny or stuffy nose, streaming and itching eyes, are also the symptoms of other allergies like dust, animal fur, etc.

To cure the tendency to hayfever, will require constitutional treatment by an experienced practitioner. The following remedies will help to alleviate discomfort without the unpleasant side effects found with hayfever drug treatment.

(See also: ALLERGIES.)

HERBS

Internal

Echinacea, Elderflower, Eyebright, Hyssop: Combine in equal quantities and make an infusion using one teaspoon per cupful of boiling water. Drink three cups per day.

External

Chamomile, Eyebright: Make an infusion as above, but cool, and then use to bathe the eyes regularly.

HOMOEOPATHY

Allium Cepa, Euphrasia, Sabadilla 6: A combination remedy that may be taken three times a day when hayfever symptoms are present.

Euphrasia Tincture: Add three to four drops to a little cooled, boiled water and bathe the eyes regularly.

AROMATHERAPY

Eucalyptus, Hyssop: Put two drops of each in a bowl of hot water and use as a steam inhalation.

HEADACHES

Nearly everyone has a headache at one time or another as there are so many causes. They may be a sign that one is over-stressed, or they may result from toxins, e.g. tobacco, alcohol, etc., or they may be associated with a cold, fever, PMT, or caused by structural conditions such as a neck injury or bad posture. Obviously, if headaches are very severe or persist, or result from an injury, medical advice must be sought immediately, because there are other more serious causes of headaches.

Alexander Technique will be useful if bad posture is a causative factor; acupuncture, homoeopathy and other therapies will help as constitutional treatment for recurrent headaches. For the occasional headache with an obvious, non-serious cause, the following remedies will be helpful.

(See also: HANGOVERS, MIGRAINE, SUNSTROKE.)

HERBS

Balm, Meadowsweet, Peppermint, Rosemary, Vervain: Combine, make an infusion using a heaped teaspoon to a cupful of boiling water, and drink a cup every few hours. Also consider the following herbs by looking them up in a herbal repertory: *Chamomile, Lady's Slipper, Lavender, Lime Flowers, Scullcap, White Willow, Wood Betony.*

HOMOEOPATHY

Aconite 6 or 30: Sudden violent headache, worse in the evening. Comes on after taking a cold or a fright.
Arnica 30: Brought on by a fall or injury. Bruised feeling in head.
Belladonna 6 or 30: Throbbing pain. Head feels hot. Dilated pupils.
Bryonia 6 or 30: Bursting, heavy, crushing, splitting headache. Worse for any movement, better lying still.
Calc Phos, Kali Phos, Mag Phos 6X: Headaches from stress, strain and overworking. One dose every two hours.
Gelsemium 6 or 30: Begins at the back of the neck. Heavy, dull headache. Associated with fluey symptoms or apprehension.

Iris 6 or 30: Aches begin with blurring of vision. Sick headaches. Shooting pain in temples. Tired headache after mental work.

Kali Bich 6 or 30: Preceded by visual disturbances. Aching in the sinuses. Pain as of a solid block in the forehead. Catarrhal headaches.

Nux Vomica 6 or 30: Irritable headache brought on by over-indulgence in coffee, alcohol, etc., or by over-studying. Overall sick feeling.

Pulsatilla 6 or 30: Headache with nausea and gastric or menstrual disturbances. Better by walking in open air. Miserable and weepy.

AROMATHERAPY

Chamomile, Eucalyptus, Lavender, Rose, Rosemary: Choose from the above, dilute in vegetable oil and massage into the temples, or for a whole body massage. Alternatively, add a few drops to a warm bath.

HIGH BLOOD PRESSURE (HYPERTENSION)

There are many factors involved in this common problem, and prevention is much better than cure. A holistic practitioner should be consulted to look into the main contributing aspects in each case. Ongoing supervision is crucial: once recognised, regular checks over an indefinite period should be arranged with a physician. Many people need to continue lifelong with treatment in order to prevent stroke, kidney disease or heart failure.

A diet rich in animal fats, salt and simple sugars should be avoided, as should smoking and alcohol consumption. A high-stress lifestyle is also a predisposing factor. Sometimes the problem is hereditary.

HERBS

If taking hypertension drugs, a qualified herbalist must be consulted before trying herbal treatment.

Hawthorn, Lime Flowers, Mistletoe, Yarrow: This mixture may be helpful for mild cases. Combine the herbs and make an infusion using one heaped teaspoon of herbs to a cupful of boiling water and stand for ten minutes before straining. Drink a cupful twice daily for up to six weeks.

HOMOEOPATHY

Constitutional treatment is advised. The following homoeo-pathic tinctures may be of benefit.

Cactus, China, Crataegus: A combination of tinctures that acts as a circulation tonic. Five drops in a wine glass of water three times a day.

Crataegus: Five drops in a wine glass of water three times a day.

AROMATHERAPY

Most benefit will be received from regular massage by an experienced aromatherapist.

Clary Sage, Lavender, Melissa: Regular baths containing a few drops of one of these oils may be tried.

BACH FLOWER REMEDIES®

We suggest that you look into the use of Bach Flower Remedies® to help with the stress-induced factor of this problem.

HYPERACTIVITY

Hyperactivity is a syndrome marked by sleeplessness, restless-ness and aggressive behaviour. It is not easy to diagnose because the problem varies a lot in degrees, but it does seem to be an increasing problem, particularly in children. Recent research suggests that allergies, food additives and pollution are primary factors to consider; however emotional upset due to family dynamics may also be very significant.

Constitutional treatment by a holistic practitioner is strongly recommended.

I

Golden Seal
(Hydrastis Canadensis)

IMPETIGO

A highly contagious infection often contracted from animals; appearing as sores, most commonly on the hands or face, and may include other symptoms such as loss of appetite, nausea, headache and swelling. Scrupulous hygiene is essential to avoid infection and infecting others.

HERBS

External

Echinacea, Golden Seal, Marigold, St John's Wort: Use equal parts to make a decoction and bathe regularly.

Internal

Echinacea, Poke Root: Use equal parts, make a decoction and drink three times daily.

HOMOEOPATHY

External

Hypercal Tincture: Add three or four drops of the tincture to a little cool, boiled water and bathe frequently.

Internal

Ant. Crude 6: Oozing eruptions with thick yellow crusts. Worse on face; individual sores joining together. Looks worse after bathing. Three doses a day for ten days.

Ars Alb 6: Sores bleed, with burning pains and rawness, better from warmth. Exudes a thin watery fluid. Three doses a day for ten days.

Graphites 6: Scabby oozing eruptions with sticky discharge. Three doses a day for ten days.

Merc Sol 6: Deep open sores with yellowish crusts exuding offensive smelling pus. Three doses a day for ten days.

Rhus Tox 6: Extremely itchy and burning sores, blister-like eruptions. Three doses a day for ten days.

AROMATHERAPY

Lavender, Marigold (Tagetes), Patchouli, Tea Tree, Thyme: Use one of these oils in a steam bath.

INCONTINENCE

This is most common in the elderly, and the chronically sick. If there is no organic problem involved other than loss of control in the sphincter muscle of the bladder, or nervous debility, the following suggestions may be helpful.

(See also: BEDWETTING.)

HERBS

Agrimony, Bayberry, Horsetail: Make an infusion of two parts *Horsetail* to one part *Agrimony* and drink a cupful two or three times daily as a tonic for the urinary system.

HOMOEOPATHY

Causticum 30: Bedwetting during first sleep at night. Stress incontinence. Paralysis and weakness of bladder. No sensation in urethra when passing urine. Two doses eight hours apart. May be repeated after six weeks.

Equisetum 6: Habitual bedwetting with fullness and distension in bladder. Dribbling urine in the elderly. One dose morning and night for ten days.

Sepia 30: Loss of tone of pelvic area and sphincter muscles. Stress incontinence after labour. Two doses eight hours apart. May be repeated after six weeks.

INDIGESTION

The digestive system may be upset by the intake of rich food, or by the person eating when feeling stressful or tense, or due to fast or irregular eating. The symptoms include heartburn, nausea, flatulence and general discomfort in the stomach region. Occasional dyspeptic symptoms will be felt by most people sometimes, but if the problem is more persistant or constitutes a marked change from a previously stable pattern, professional advice should be sought, because indigestion can be an early symptom of several different digestive diseases.
(See also: GASTRITIS.)

HERBS

Aniseed, Cardamon, Fennel: A few of any of these seeds chewed after a meal will help with indigestion.

Balm, Peppermint, Vervain: A tea made from any of these will be soothing for the digestive system. Drink after a meal.

Meadowsweet: Combine this with any of the teas mentioned above if symptoms of acidity are also present.

HOMOEOPATHY

Ars Alb 6: Irritable stomach. Burning in stomach area. Great thirst for hot drinks. Anxious, restless patient. One every two to three hours.

Carbo Veg 6: Distension and heaviness. Sour, disordered

89

stomach. Flatulence, belching, heartburn and waterbrash. All food turns to wind. Particularly useful in elderly patients. Two or three doses four hours apart.

Kali Mur 6X: Heavy feeling. Coated, white tongue. Indigestion after rich, fatty food. One dose every few hours.

Nat Phos 6X: Sour risings, heartburn. Liverish symptoms. Acidity. One dose every few hours.

Nux Vom 6: Heartburn, belching. Weight and pain in stomach. Brought on by over-indulgence of food and drink. Irritable. One dose every few hours as necessary.

Pulsatilla 6: From eating fatty food. Nausea. Feeling of distension. Unpleasant taste in the mouth. Better in fresh air. Thirstless. One dose every few hours.

AROMATHERAPY

Cardamon, Fennel, Peppermint: Add a few drops of the above to a vegetable based oil and massage into the stomach area.

INFLUENZA

Influenza commonly called 'flu' is an acute infection of the respiratory tract similar to colds, but more severe, and accompanied by symptoms like fever, aches and coughs. Different strains will produce different symptoms, e.g., sore throat, nausea, and these should be treated specifically. Flu normally lasts between two and five days, but more serious complications may develop, particularly in the elderly. Persons not responding to treatment should be referred to a practitioner. It seems that an increasing trend with 'flu' is to leave the person debilitated and depressed.

(See also: COLDS, CONVALESCENCE.)

HERBS

Boneset, Elderflower, Peppermint: A general mixture. Combine, infuse, and drink several times a day. The following herbs may also be added to this mixture.

Echinacea, Poke Root: If symptoms linger.

Elderflower, Peppermint and Composition Mixture: An easy to use effective flu remedy. Take two teaspoons in hot water three times daily.

Pleurisy Root: If a cough is present.

Red Sage: If accompanied by a sore throat.

Vervain: If accompanied by depression.

HOMOEOPATHY

Aconite 30: Sudden onset with fever. Dry, painful cough. Restlessness and anxiety; symptoms develop after exposure to cold winds. Two doses on first day of symptoms.

Ars Alb 6 or 30: Shivering, restlessness, anxiety; loss of appetite; desires hot drinks; worse from cold drinks. Burning sensations; worse after midnight. Feels very chilly. Take three doses of the 6th potency a day for five days, or one dose of the 30th potency a day for three days.

Bryonia 6 or 30: Worse with movement; desire to be alone; irritable; dry and thirsty; painful cough, throat and chest. Take three doses of the 6th potency a day for five days, or one dose of the 30th potency a day for three days.

Eupatorium Perf 6 or 30: Intense aching; bursting headache; soreness of eyeballs. Hacking cough and hoarseness; nausea; marked thirst. Take three doses of the 6th potency a day for five days, or one dose of the 30th potency a day for three days.

Gelsemium 6 or 30: Heaviness, and drowsy patient; chills up and down the spine. Aching in limbs and head. Little thirst. General flu symptoms. Take three doses of the 6th potency a day for five days, or one dose of the 30th potency a day for three days.

Rhus Tox 6 or 30: Extremely restless, muscles stiff and aching. Chill; worse after getting cold or wet. Thirsty, hoarseness. Take three doses of the 6th potency a day for five days, or one dose of the 30th potency a day for three days.

AROMATHERAPY

Benzoin, Lavender, Rosemary: Dilute in suitable vegetable oil base and massage into chest and aching limbs.

Eucalyptus: Add a few drops to hot water. Use as a steam inhalation for congestion.

INSOMNIA

Sleeplessness may be a short-term or long-term problem. The amount of sleep needed will vary from person to person, and for the same person at different stages of their life. Short-term sleeplessness may be brought about by anxiety, fear, stress or excitement. Most people will suffer the odd sleepless night at some time; the problem is that sleeplessness can become rather a habit, and anxiety will develop around not being able to sleep which may become self-perpetuating. Sleep disorders such as early morning waking, if accompanied by dark moods, can indicate an underlying depression which may need professional help. The following remedies will be useful to break the habit, but for chronic insomniacs constitutional treatment by a qualified practitioner will be necessary.

A useful exercise if the mind is full of thoughts and unresolved problems is to mentally work backwards through the day going over everything you have done without becoming attached to any one issue. Stimulating foods and drinks, and eating late at night can all be aggravating factors, and should be avoided.

HERBS

Balm, Chamomile, Lime Flowers, Orange Blossom, Passiflora: A pleasant tasting relaxing bedtime drink.

Scullcap, Vervain: Add these to the above mixture if nervous tension is present.

Valerian: Add if the mixture needs to be stronger, e.g. if pain is present. This particular herb does not suit everybody, and may become habit-forming, so do not use too frequently.

HOMOEOPATHY

Aconite 6: Anxiety with restlessness and fear. Anxious dreams. Two or three doses at 30 minute intervals.

Arnica 6: Sleeplessness due to being overtired, after overworking, or due to shock. Body aches and the bed feels too hard. Two or three doses.

Coffea 6: Thoughts racing around the mind. Sleeplessness due to anxiety and agitation. Two or three doses at 30 minute intervals.

Kali Phos 6X: Nervous tension, habitual sleeplessness. Take one a night for ten nights; this remedy should begin to work after the second or third night.

Kali Phos, Mag Phos, Nat Phos 6X: Aids sleep after stress. Insomnia from being under strain and overwrought. Two or three doses at 30 minute intervals.

Nux Vomica 30: Person falls asleep in the evening, but wakes too early and still feels tired when it is time to get up. Irritability. Indigestion. Try one dose and do not repeat for several weeks.

AROMATHERAPY

Chamomile, Lavender, Neroli, Rose: Add a few drops of the above mixture to a warm bath.

Lavender: Put a couple of drops on a piece of cotton cloth and place on the pillow.

BACH FLOWER REMEDIES®

The following may be useful when dealing with the emotional contributory factors.

Olive: Exhaustion, tired but sleepless. Needing sleep.

Vervain: Over-straining, over-enthusiasm.

White Chestnut: Persistant and racing worries and troubles.

Oat
(Avena sativa)

JET LAG

There are a few remedies which may ease the discomfort often felt during or after travelling by air. Symptoms are due to a combination of sitting or sleeping for long periods of time where the circulation is impeded, the body struggling to become accustomed to the time changes and change of sleep patterns and, thirdly, to the changing pressure in the aircraft. Avoid alcohol as this will add to the dehydration resulting from the pressure changes; drink plenty of spring water.

HERBS

Oat Tincture: A mildly diuretic nervine tincture to be taken during the flight to ease swelling in the feet and aid relaxation. Ten drops in water every six hours.

Kola, Oat, Rosemary Tinctures: This mixture will stimulate and tonify the nervous system and help you to adjust on arrival. Buy as a mixture and take ten drops in water every four to six hours during the flight.

HOMOEOPATHY

AAA 30: Fear and anticipation of the flight. One dose the previous day and one before take-off.

Kali Mur 6 or 30: Earache due to pressure changes. One dose before take-off, and take as necessary.

Kali Phos 6X: A nerve tonic for exhaustion, sleeplessness and tension. Take every six hours on board and for two to three days after arrival as required.

Nat Mur 6X: To encourage the body to maintain correct water distribution, prevents dehydration. One dose every four hours.

AROMATHERAPY

Rosemary: A few drops on your handkerchief inhaled at regular intervals; or take a *Rosemary* bath on arrival adding three to four drops to the bath water.

L

Daisy
(Bellis perennis)

LABOUR

The progress of the birth of a child, of which there are three stages: (1) dilatation of the cervix; (2) the passage of the foetus through the canal, and the birth; and (3) from the birth of the child to the expulsion of the placenta.

Childbirth is a natural process; there are many books available to help prepare yourself and your environment. The following remedies may complement the aid and advice of a competent midwife and/or doctor. It is advisable to be under the guidance of a qualified practitioner during pregnancy, and they should be able to advise you on your labour.

(See also: PREGNANCY.)

HERBS

Raspberry Leaf, Squaw Vine: Can be drunk during the last three months of pregnancy to help facilitate labour.

HOMOEOPATHY

Aconite 30 or 200: Fear, shock, after pains with fear and restlessness. One or two doses.

Arnica 30 or 200: Bruising and symptoms of over-exhaustion

96

after labour. One dose on first going into labour, and one a day for a couple of days after. Promotes healing.

Carbo Veg 30; Exhaustion during long labour, craves fresh air. One or two doses.

Caulophyllum 30 or 200: Labour pains are weak or irregular, or may cease from exhaustion. One or two doses.

Gelsemium 30: Rigid or nervous fear and trembling during early stages of labour. One or two doses.

Mag Phos 30: Shooting, stabbing after-pains. One or two doses.

Pulsatilla 30: Weak labour pains. Patient feels irritable and weepy, craves fresh air; after-pains too long and too violent. One or two doses.

AROMATHERAPY

Clary Sage: Can be burned or sprayed in the room to freshen it.

Jasmine: To help with the pain of childbirth; massaged on the lower back in a base of vegetable oil.

Rose: Is cooling and soothing. Can be used diluted in a vegetable base oil for massage.

BACH FLOWER REMEDIES®

Rescue Remedy®: If the labour is long and exhausting, and if there is fear or panic involved. Take as necessary.

LABOUR (POST)

HERBS

External

Comfrey, Horsetail, Marigold, St John's Wort: Add one heaped tablespoonful to a pint of water. Leave to infuse and pour into a warm bath for a soothing and healing effect to the perineum.

Internal

Raspberry Leaf, Squaw Vine: Encourages the uterus to return back to normal. Make an infusion using a heaped teaspoon to a cup of boiling water. Drink two times daily for two or three weeks.

Blue Cohosh: If after-pains are present. Make a docoction and drink three times a day.

Nettle, Red Clover: If exhaustion is present. Make an infusion and drink a cupful twice daily.

HOMOEOPATHY

Bellis Perennis 30: Painful, sensitive feeling in genital organs after forceps delivery, or pain in abdomen after Caesarian birth. Two doses a day for three days.

Calendula 30: To heal episiotomy or lacerations during forceps delivery. Two doses a day for four days.

Chamomilla 30: Severe after-pains, patient is acutely sensitive to pain, feels irritable. Two or three doses over two days.

Hypercal Tincture: Useful after an episiotomy or tear. Dilute a few drops in a cup of water and bathe area.

Mag Phos 30: Spasmodic shooting after-pains. Two or three doses over two days.

AROMATHERAPY

Marigold (Tagetes), Lavender: For soothing baths after child-birth, dilute in a dispersing base and add to a warm bath.

LIVER PROBLEMS

The liver is the largest organ of the body, and is involved either directly or indirectly in all physiological processes. One of its important functions is in the eliminating process of toxins, and thus a diet including chemicals, additives, alcohol or drugs will place strain on the liver. It is often helpful to aid the liver with a cleansing diet and purifying herbs, even if no symptoms of liver disease are present; and most spring cleansing remedies and diets contain liver detoxifiers. There are many symptoms of liver disease; including constipation, nausea, sluggishness, irritability, poor skin, pain in the liver region and dull headaches. If you suspect there is any actual disease of the liver, consult a qualified practitioner. Avoid fatty, rich foods, alcohol and coffee. The following remedies will be cleansing and tonifying.

HERBS

Balmony, Burdock, Centaury, Dandelion, Nettle: Combine equal quantities and make an infusion using one teaspoon per cup. Drink three cups per day.

HOMOEOPATHY

Nat Phos 6X: Liverishness, acidity, poor digestion, sour risings. Twice a day for ten days.
Nat Sulph 6X: Heaviness, sluggishness, bilious vomiting. Twice a day for ten days.

AROMATHERAPY

Grapefruit, Juniper, Rosemary: These oils will help detoxify the liver. Use in a massage base oil or add to a warm bath.

LARYNGITIS

(See: SORE THROATS.)

M

Bryony~(Bryonia alba)

MASTITIS

Inflammation of the breasts. This may be due to infection (most common when breastfeeding), growths, or part of a pre-menstrual picture, and thus may be either acute or of a chronic nature. If symptoms are persistent, a qualified practitioner must be seen for a diagnosis and treatment. For pre-menstrual mastitis, try *Evening Primrose Oil Capsules*, two a day for ten days before each period. It is advisable for all women to perform monthly self-examination so that any deviation from the norm can be noted and checked out by a competent practitioner.

There is some evidence that caffeine may aggravate the tendency to cystic growth formation in the breasts, and thus tea and coffee should be avoided. The following remedies may be tried for acute mastitis. If symptoms persist consult medical advice.

(See also: BREASTFEEDING.)

HERBS

External

Comfrey, Marshmallow, Slippery Elm: These herbs can be used to make a soothing poultice for acute mastitis.

Internal

Echinacea, Marigold, Poke Root, Wild Yam: Combine, make a decoction and drink three times a day for acute inflammation.

HOMOEOPATHY

Belladonna 6 or 30: Pain, throbbing and redness in breast. Streaks radiate from the nipple. Breast feels heavy and hard. One dose every few hours until pain diminishes.

Bryonia 6 or 30: Breast hot, painful and hard. Cannot bear touch or movement. Better for hard pressure or keeping still. Undue engorgement of breasts. One dose every few hours until improvement occurs.

Phytolacca 6 or 30: Heavy, stony hard, swollen or tender breasts, pain during breastfeeding or worse before menses. Nipples cracked and sensitive. One dose every few hours until improvement occurs.

AROMATHERAPY

Chamomile, Geranium, Peppermint, Rose: Dilute a few drops of each in water. Apply as a soothing and cooling compress.

Lavender: This oil diluted in the bath will be soothing.

Essential oils are too strong for a baby, so the breasts must be washed free from the oil before the baby feeds again.

MEASLES

An infectious disease common in children; the incubation period is ten to twelve days. Early symptoms are those of a cold, sore throat, inflamed eyes, cough, rise in temperature, and possibly you may be able to see 'Koplik's spots' (small, white spots on the inside of the cheeks).

The rash appears on about the fourth day on the neck and behind the ears, gradually extending to the rest of the body and extremities. Recovery usually occurs by about the seventh or ninth day. The most infectious period is before the rash appears.

The disease is not usually dangerous, but complications can develop; usually due to a high fever with dehydration, or breathing difficulties due to chest infection. Rarely, a more serious complication involving inflammation of the brain tissues — encephalitis — may occur: any unusual drowsiness or irritability should be assessed by a medical practitioner. The eyes may also become sore and inflamed, and the rash may cause distress from itching. If any symptoms are very marked or persistent, seek immediate professional advice. Antibiotics do not have any effect on the virus, so they should not be prescribed unless complications set in.

We do not recommend innoculation against measles because the long-term effects of this are not known, and we believe, as with all childhood illnesses, measles provides the opportunity for the child to strengthen his/her vitality and throw off miasmatic tendencies.

General home care should involve bed rest in a darkened room, and during the fever sponging down with tepid water.

HERBS

Internal

Boneset, Chamomile, Echinacea, Elderflowers, Yarrow: Make an infusion of a combination of these herbs using one teaspoon of herbs to a cupful of boiling water. Stand for ten minutes, then strain and drink a cupful three times a day.

External

Eyebright: Make an infusion and when cool, strain and bathe the eyes with the solution to soothe them.
Chamomile, Marigold, Marshmallow: Combine the herbs and make an infusion using one tablespoon of herbs to a pint of boiling water. When cool, strain and use the solution to sponge down the body to cool down feverishness and soothe irritation or itching.

HOMOEOPATHY

Aconite 6 or 30: For initial stages. Restless, fearful child, high temperature, eyes ache with light. Eyes and nose streaming, hard croupy cough. Give every few hours until improvement occurs.

Belladonna 30 or 200: Restless, flushed, high temperature and delirium, sore throat, disturbed by noise, light and movement. One or two doses.

Bryonia 6 or 30: Use if the rash is slow to appear; accompanied by painful, dry cough; thirsty; irritable; worse from movement. Two or three doses a day.

Euphrasia 6 or 30: Marked eye symptoms and nasal discharge. Eyes watery, sore and inflamed. Acrid tears, harsh cough, throbbing headache. Two or three doses over two days.

Kali Bich 6 or 30; Laryngitis with hoarse, brassy cough, cough predominates, earache and nausea, eyes water and eyelids stick together. Two or three doses over two to three days.

Morbillinum 30: For cases not responding to treatment, this is the measles nosode. One dose only.

Pulsatilla 6 or 30: Catarrhal symptoms; profuse lachrymation; cough dry at night, looser in daytime; dry mouth, but seldom thirsty. Two or three doses over two to three days.

AROMATHERAPY

Chamomile, Eucalyptus, Lavender: Dilute a few drops in water and use to sponge down the body.

MENOPAUSE

A time of transition when the ovaries stop releasing an ovum every month, and the woman is no longer fertile. Menstruation stops because there is no stimulus from the ovaries.

The age of the menopause varies although it is generally from the middle or later forties. The onset can be gradual with the periods coming less frequently, or it may occur quite suddenly.

Reactions to the menopause seem to depend on the general state of health and on the ability to cope with transition. In physical terms the accompanying changes are due to a re-adjustment of pituitary and ovarian hormones. The most commonly experienced problematic symptoms are hot flushes, palpitations, nervous irritability, depression and general debil-ity. Many of the symptoms blamed on the menopause are not due to it; and there is a real danger of neglecting other disorders that could and should be treated. Any post menopausal vaginal bleeding should be assessed by a medical practitioner.

This is a time when constitutional treatment, e.g. by an acupuncturist, herbalist or homoeopath, and emotional support e.g. from support groups, can make a tremendous difference to making the transition a positive time of change.

Any persistent discomfort, particularly heavy menstrual bleeding for more than two or three periods, and any inter-menstrual bleeding, should be referred to a qualified practi-tioner. Hormonal replacement will delay the symptoms rather than encourage the body to adjust as well as having the risk of side-effects.

HERBS

Agnus Castus, False Unicorn, Hops, St John's Wort, Wild Yam, Yarrow: A useful mixture to help the body make its hormonal adjustments and tonify the reproductive system. Make a decoction and drink twice a day for six weeks.

Blackcurrant Leaves, Hawthorn Tops, Sage: Add these herbs if there are hot flushes.

St John's Wort, Skullcap, Vervain, Wild Oat: Add these herbs if nervousness or depression is marked.

HOMOEOPATHY

Constitutional treatment by a qualified homoeopath can be of great benefit to help with the physical and mental symptoms associated with the menopause.

AROMATHERAPY

A course of treatment by an experienced aromatherapist, who can select oils for your specific needs, will be of most benefit.
Geranium, Rose: These oils will help to balance hormones and tone the uterus. Apply in a bath on a regular basis.

BACH FLOWER REMEDIES®

Look through the list to find the remedies needed for your particular symptoms. We especially suggest:
Impatiens: Nervous irritability and impatience.
Olive: For weakness, weariness and tiredness.
Walnut: To help with times of transition and change.

MENSTRUAL PROBLEMS

Pain, frequency and duration of menses will vary from woman to woman, and for the same woman at different stages of her life, and to a great extent will reflect her general state of health.

Problems may arise due to hormonal, psychological, mechanical damage, cysts, fibroids, tumours, circulatory or nutritional factors. In any case it is important to assess which factors are most significant. Any problem which becomes severely uncomfortable or is persistent should be referred to a qualified practitioner. This is particularly true if inter-menstrual bleeding occurs, or there are any signs of infection, e.g. pain, unpleasant discharge or increased temperature.

The most common menstrual ailment we are asked to treat is painful periods. Pain at the start of a period is vaguely ascribed to reduction of blood-flow by spasm of the uterus, and pain that comes on later to congestion. We suggest that the following remedies may be helpful in treating painful periods, and as tonics for the reproductive system. Periods which cease or become markedly irregular or heavy require constitutional treatment, because this is a longer-term situation that is not

105

really within the scope of self-diagnosis and treatment.
(See also: MENOPAUSE, PRE-MENSTRUAL TENSION.)

HERBS

Agnus Castus, False Unicorn, Motherwort, Squaw Vine: Herbs to
tonify the uterus and balance the hormones. Combine and
drink three times a day for six weeks.
Chamomile, Cramp Bark, Marigold, Passiflora, Raspberry: For
period pains. Combine and drink three times a day when
required.
Shepherd's Purse: Add this herb if bleeding is heavy.

HOMOEOPATHY

Aconite 30: Menses suppressed due to fright, shock or after
exposure to cold. One dose at bedtime, and one the
following morning.
Apis 6 or 30: Burning, stinging pains during or before menses.
Scanty discharge of blood. Patient is hot and thirstless. One
dose every few hours as required.
Belladonna 6 or 30: Menses early and profuse. Violent bearing
down and throbbing pains. Throbbing headache. One dose
every few hours as necessary.
Bryonia 6 or 30: Menses early and profuse. Cutting pains in
uterus and breasts. Splitting headache. Everything is worse
for motion and better keeping still and applying pressure.
One dose every few hours as required.
Mag Phos 6X: Cramping, shooting and spasmodic pains. Pains
are better for warmth and rubbing. Dissolve a couple of pills
in hot water and sip as required, or dissolve one dose under
the tongue every few hours.

AROMATHERAPY

*Chamomile, Clary Sage, Cypress, Marigold (Tagetes), Marjoram,
Rose:* Choose two or three oils from the above and add a few
drops of each to a vegetable oil base and massage into the
abdomen to soothe pain. Or add two or three drops to one
of the above for a soothing warm bath.

MIGRAINE

Migraine is distinguished from a headache by its intensity; it is often accompanied by nausea and vision disorders and usually affects one side of the head. The pain is produced by spasm of blood vessels in the brain. The length of the attack varies from a couple of hours to several days. Effective treatment must be constitutional as the causes are so varied. Contributory factors include stress, tension, hormonal cycles in women, congestive disorders, allergic reactions, and a hereditary pre-disposition.

We feel that individuals can go a long way in helping themselves treat this ailment by ascertaining the more profound reasons why they are the victims, and then as far as possible reducing the factors that stimulate them. Psychotherapy may be useful for this approach.

If the migraine attacks are mild or infrequent, here are some remedies to try.

HERBS

Balm, Feverfew, Meadowsweet, Rosemary: Combine the above herbs, make an infusion and drink up to three cups a day.
Scullcap: Add this herb if nervous tension is present.

HOMOEOPATHY

Belladonna 6 or 30: Intense and violent throbbing pains. Sensitive to noise or movement. Pain begins suddenly, focused on forehead. Headache relieved by sitting down. Two or three doses.
Bryonia 6 or 30: Worse from movement, relieved by pressure. Heavy, crushing pain may be accompanied by nausea and vomiting. Patient thirsty and irritable.
Gelsemium 6 or 30; Headaches begin at the back of the head, preceded by visual disturbances. Pain extends like a band around the head. Dull, heavy headaches, patient feels

confused. Better after urination. Two or three doses.

Nux Vomica 6 or 30: Headache brought on by overeating or use of stimulants; accompanied by overall sick feeling. Worse for cold air or wind. Worse in morning. Patient very irritable. Two or three doses.

Pulsatilla 6 or 30: Associated with digestive upsets, menstrual periods or emotional upsets. Pain in forehead accompanied by throbbing. Better from open air. Nausea. Patient feels weepy. Two or three doses.

AROMATHERAPY

Basil, Marjoram, Melissa, Rose: Choose one of the above. Dilute a few drops in almond oil and massage into temples.

MISCARRIAGE

The first symptom of a miscarriage (spontaneous abortion), is bleeding, sometimes accompanied with pain. It is thought that many miscarriages occur as the body's natural way of rejecting an unhealthy foetus. Thus, no form of treatment should be taken to prevent a miscarriage at all costs. However, miscarriage can also be threatened in case of weakness, stress or trauma in the pregnant woman and then the appropriate remedies may be taken to avoid an unnecessary miscarriage.

Plenty of rest is necessary in all cases of threatened miscarriage. Having excluded other causes of bleeding (e.g. ectopic pregnancy), care should be supervised by a competent medical practitioner who should be kept informed of any changes in the patient's condition.

The emotional trauma experienced after a miscarriage can be considerable, and in this case the support of an experienced and caring practitioner would be a helpful adjunct to that of friends and family.

If there is a history of miscarriages, constitutional treatment will be necessary from the outset of pregnancy, or before. Here we can only offer remedies that may help in conjunction with

treatment from a qualified holistic practitioner.
(See also: PREGNANCY.)

HERBS

For herbs that must be avoided during pregnancy, see
PREGNANCY.
Cramp Bark, False Unicorn, Wild Yam: A useful uterine tonic to
take if a miscarriage is threatening. Combine the herbs,
make a decoction by simmering a teaspoon of herbs in a
mugful of water for ten minutes, and drink a cupful three
times a day. Alternatively combine the tinctures, and take
one teaspoonful in a wine glass of water three times a day.
Scullcap: If there is considerable stress involved this herb can
be added.

HOMOEOPATHY

Aconite 30 or 200: Miscarriage threatens suddenly, usually
following a fright, shock or trauma. Marked fearfulness and
anxiety. One or two doses.
Arnica 30 or 200: Miscarriage threatens after an accident or
trauma. Haemorrhage following a blow or accident. Haemorrhage after intercourse. One or two doses.
Chamomilla 30 or 200: Threatening miscarriage with distressing,
contractive pains. Loss of dark blood with the occasional
gush of bright red blood. Symptoms may come on after
anger. One or two doses.
Pulsatilla 30 or 200: Changeable symptoms. Patient is weepy
and in need of support. Malposition of foetus. One or two
doses only.
Sepia 30 or 200: Weak, dragging or bearing down sensation in
the uterus. Patient is tired and irritable. One or two doses.

AROMATHERAPY

A course of tonifying massage after a miscarriage will help the
body to recover more quickly. Consult an experienced
aromatherapist.

If there is any predisposition to miscarriage, all essential oils
should be avoided in the early months of pregnancy.

109

BACH FLOWER REMEDIES®

Rescue Remedy®: For fear, shock and anguish. Take a few drops as required.

For the emotional after effects of a miscarriage, or for fear of a miscarriage, consult the list in the appendix, or look through a more detailed book on the Bach Flower Remedies® and select the most appropriate remedies.

MISCARRIAGE — ABORTION (AFTER EFFECTS)

A deliberately induced termination of pregnancy usually before sixteen weeks.

Consideration should be given to the need for ongoing emotional support and possible psychotherapy. Be cautious about the possibility of any infection following an abortion: if suspected, seek urgent medical attention.

HERBS

Blue Cohosh, False Unicorn, Holy Thistle, Liquorice, Sarsaparilla: A tea to balance hormones and retone the uterus. Combine the herbs and make a decoction using one teaspoon of herbs to a mugful of water and simmer for ten minutes. Strain and drink a cupful three times a day for two weeks.
Scullcap, Valerian: These may be added to the above mixture if there is a considerable amount of stress involved.

HOMOEOPATHY

Arnica 200: For shock and bruising. Will also help to prevent haemorrhage and infection. Take one dose before the abortion and one dose afterwards.
Bellis Perennis 30: For the after effects of mechanical interference in the uterus. Bruised sensation in the abdomen. Yellow discharge. Two or three doses eight hours apart.

Ignatia 200: Grief and sadness dating from an abortion. One dose only.

Staphysagria 200: For after effects of mechanical interference in the womb, combined with unexpressed sadness and anger. One dose only.

AROMATHERAPY

Lavender, Marigold (Tagetes): Add five drops of each to the warm water for a soothing and healing bath.

Neroli, Rose: Uplifting and tonifying oils. Wear as perfume or use as a massage or in the bath.

BACH FLOWER REMEDIES®

Rescue Remedy®: For anguish, fear and shock. Take a few drops as often as required.

Look at the brief list in the Appendix of this book or study a more detailed book on the Bach Flower Remedies® to help in selecting other appropriate remedies.

MORNING SICKNESS

Symptoms include nausea, occasional vomiting and weakness. Some morning sickness is experienced by most women during the first few months of pregnancy. It is most frequently experienced in the morning, when the stomach is empty, although it may occur at any time of day. The traditional cure of eating a dry biscuit before rising is well worth trying. It seems to be caused by the massive upheaval of hormones occurring in the body, combined with low blood sugar. Symptoms usually recede after the third month of pregnancy, rarely the symptoms will persist throughout pregnancy, in which case professional help should be sought. Guidance should also be sought if vomiting is persistent, or any aversion to eating is prolonged.

Whilst it is best to avoid any medication during pregnancy,

(unless specifically advised by your practitioner), the following remedies are gentle and safe and may help with this annoying symptom. Do consult your practitioner first if you are under treatment.

HERBS

Balm, Black Horehound, Ginger, Meadowsweet, Peppermint: This is a calming and soothing tea to help with nausea and acidity. Combine one part *Balm* to two parts *Meadowsweet* and infuse, drink three times daily.

HOMOEOPATHY

Ipecac 6: Persistent nausea that is not alleviated by vomiting. One or two doses daily as required.

Nat Phos 6X: Nausea with sour risings. One or two doses as required.

Nux Vomica 6: Nausea which is ameliorated by vomiting. Sour eructations, retching, indigestion. One or two doses as required.

Pulsatilla 6: Nausea with little vomiting and improved by fresh air. One or two doses as required.

Sepia 6: Nausea aggravated by the smell or thought of food, although may be ameliorated by eating. Weak, sinking sensation in stomach. Vomiting. One or two doses as required.

AROMATHERAPY

Lavender: One drop in a warm bath, or as a warm compress applied to the abdomen. (Warm a flannel in warm water and a drop of the oil. Place on the abdomen, wrap a large towel around you to keep warm.)

If there is any predisposition to miscarriage it is advisable to avoid all essential oils in the early months of pregnancy.

MOUTH ULCERS

Painful, small blisters on gums, tongue or mouth linings which are surrounded by redness. The appearance of mouth ulcers may indicate general debility. We recommend that care is taken with diet and rest, see CONVALESCENCE. If they occur regularly, seek constitutional treatment.

HERBS

Marigold, Myrrh, Red Sage, Thyme: Mouth washes with any of the above herbs can be used either in the form of an infusion, or tinctures diluted in warm water.

HOMOEOPATHY

Borax 6: Painful ulcers. Ulcers bleed when touched. Aggravated by eating. One three times a day for five days.

Hypericum and *Calendula Tincture:* Five drops in half an inch of warm water. Use as a mouthwash regularly.

Mercurius 6: Ulcers behind the tongue. Increased salivation. Metallic taste in mouth. Pain aggravated by heat and cold. One morning and night for five days.

Nat Phos 6X: Ulcers with acidic symptoms present. Sores and blisters on the tip of the tongue. One three times a day for five days.

AROMATHERAPY

Myrrh: Apply undiluted to the affected parts.

MUMPS

This is a highly infectious virus affecting the glands, usually the parotids, where swelling and tenderness will be noticed on the jawline. The first symptoms are often a mild fever and sore throat. Either one or both sides will be affected.

It is one of the common childhood diseases, and provides an opportunity to throw off inherited or acquired miasmatic influences. In children it is usually quite mild, but if occurring in adults, it may cause complications affecting the testicles in men and the ovaries in women. Although this rarely occurs, professional advice should be sought.

Bed rest and plenty of fluids are recommended.

HERBS

Balm, Borage, Echinacea, Poke Root, Yarrow: Use equal quantities to make a soothing infusion which will also gently cleanse the glandular system. Drink a cupful three times a day. May be sweetened with honey.

HOMOEOPATHY

Aconite 6: Every two or three hours for first couple of days. First onset of symptoms — thirst, painful throat and fever.

Apis 30: One or two doses. Throat sore, swollen, painful, puffiness. Sharp or stinging pains. No thirst.

Belladonna 30: Two or three doses as necessary. Restless, burning. Swallowing difficult, high fever, light sensitive, throbbing pains.

Clematis 30: Swelling of glands under the jaw with throbbing pain, aggravated by touch. Painful swelling of testes. Two or three doses.

Merc Sol 30: Swelling of glands under jaw. Stitching pains to the ear on swallowing. Offensive odour from mouth; saliva increased. Feverish, thirsty. Two or three doses.

Pulsatilla 30: Swelling of glands under lower jaw or going to the testes. Bad taste in mouth. Child feels miserable and weepy, wants attention. Thirstless. Two or three doses.

AROMATHERAPY

Chamomile, Lavender: Dilute a few drops of each in water and apply as a soothing and healing compress.

Eucalyptus, Thyme: Add a few drops of each to hot water for a steam inhalation that will be decongestant and assist the body to fight infection. These oils may also be sprayed in the patient's room.

N

Passion Flower ~ (Passiflora)

NAUSEA

This can vary from a slight feeling of queasiness to an over-whelming urge to vomit. Causes of nausea can be either psychological or physiological. Refer to the appropriate cross-reference or, if nausea is persistent, seek diagnosis from a practitioner. Any form of dietary indiscretion could result in nausea. The following remedies will help with an occasional bout of nausea.

(See also: ALLERGY, ANXIETY, FOOD POISONING, HANGOVER, INDIGESTION, MIGRAINE, MORNING SICKNESS, STRESS, SUN-STROKE.)

HERBS

Balm, Chamomile, Ginger, Meadowsweet, Peppermint, Vervain: An infusion of any of these teas singly or as a combination will bring soothing relief to feelings of nausea.

Cardamon Seeds: If nausea results from eating a heavy meal, chewing a few of these seeds will bring quick amelioration.

HOMOEOPATHY

Ipecac 6 or 30: Horrid nausea not relieved by vomiting. Thirstless. Sinking sensation in the stomach. Clean tongue. One dose every few hours.

Kali Mur 6X: Nausea after eating rich or fatty foods. The tongue has a white or greyish coating. One dose every three to four hours.

Kali Phos 6X: Nausea caused by nervousness. 'All gone' sensation in the stomach. One dose every three to four hours.

Nat Phos 6X: Nausea with sour risings. Brought on after eating fruit or acid food. Yellow coating to tongue. One dose every three to four hours.

Nat Sulph 6X: Nausea with bilious symptoms. Brought on after eating fatty food. Bitter taste in the mouth. Greenish coating to tongue. One dose every three to four hours.

Nux Vom 6 or 30: Nausea brought on from over-indulgence in food or alcohol. Nausea relieved by vomiting. Feels irritable. One dose every few hours.

AROMATHERAPY

Cardamom, Fennel, Ginger, Melissa, Peppermint: A few drops of either of these oils in a little vegetable oil and massaged into the stomach area will relieve feelings of nausea.

NEURALGIA

Neuralgia is a painful condition originating from an inflamed nerve. The most common sites are the trigeminal nerves in the face, and the sciatic nerve which causes pain in the lower back and thighs. A fortifying diet with particular attention to additional B complex vitamins will help this condition.

HERBS

Oats, Passiflora, St John's Wort, Scullcap: These herbs are nervine tonics. Combine and make an infusion using one teaspoon per cup, drink three cupfuls a day.

117

HOMOEOPATHY

Calc Phos 6X: Use afterwards as a nerve restorative. Morning and night for ten days.

Ferrum Phos 6X: Acute neuralgic pains due to inflammation, caused by chills, fever, etc. One dose three times a day.

Hypericum 6 or 30: Tingling, burning and numbness, worse after injury, or caused by injury. Very severe nerve pain. Either one 30 potency a day for three days or one 6 potency three times a day for five days.

Kali Phos 6X: A nerve nutrient, restlessness, exhaustion and neuralgic pain. May be taken in alternation with *Mag Phos*. Two doses a day for ten days.

Mag Phos 6X: Shooting, spasmodic neuralgic pains aggravated by cold. Alternate with *Kali Phos*. Two doses daily for ten days.

Spigelia 30: Trigeminal neuralgia with violent burning and stitching pains radiating outwards. Worse for touch. One dose a day for three days.

AROMATHERAPY

Chamomile, Marjoram, Rosemary, Sandalwood: Used in a light vegetable base oil for a local massage or compress. Also combined, or used separately, adding three to four drops to a warm bath as often as required.

NOSEBLEEDS

This may occur as a result of injury to the nose, or sometimes from disorders of the blood. If the delicate veins inside the nose are damaged by a previous accident, then even a trivial knock to the area will trigger off a nosebleed.

In children, nosebleeds are very common. If an adult suddenly develops recurring nosebleeds, then professional advice should be sought.

A course of *Rutin* tablets will help strengthen the vein walls if nosebleeds are frequent. First-aid measures include pinching the nose or placing an ice-cold compress on the back of the neck for a few minutes until the bleeding ceases.

HERBS

St Johns Wort, Witchazel, Yarrow: These are astringents to encourage the bleeding to stop. Make an infusion to saturate a piece of cotton wool and hold under the nose.

HOMOEOPATHY

Aconite 6 or 30: Nosebleed triggered by a shock or fright. One or two doses.

Arnica 6 or 30: Nosebleed after injury or trauma to the nose. Nosebleed after a fit of coughing. One or two doses.

Ferrum Phos 6X: Bright red blood. Nosebleeds in children. One or two doses.

Phosphorus 6 or 30: Nosebleeds in nervous types. Bright blood slow to stop. One or two doses.

AROMATHERAPY

Cypress: A few drops of essential oil applied to cotton wool and held under the nose for a few moments will arrest bleeding.

O

Yellow Jasmine
(Gelsemium sempervivens)

OBESITY

A condition arising from excess of fat, generally brought about by overeating, or eating the wrong foods. Often psychological or cultural factors determine our opinions on what is a fat person and what isn't. We feel that the correct weight for a person is very individual; based on the optimum efficiency of the body. This is creating a balance between two opposites — a weakness brought about by being underweight, and sluggishness and other problems arising from fatness.

Too many carbohydrates alongside insufficient exercise produces fat which stays in the body. Fat people run a greater risk of ill-health, including heart and circulation problems and diseases of the kidneys.

Reducing fat in the body can really only be brought about naturally by eating less carbohydrates and increasing the output of energy. Slimming, or rather weight reduction, requires common sense in both psychological and nutritional terms. Counselling alongside diet control is advisable. Evidence suggests that a balanced wholefood diet is preferable; consult a naturopath or other natural physicians for advice.

OPERATIONS (PREPARATION AND AFTER EFFECTS)

Post-operational distress and depression can be somewhat alleviated by supplementing the diet with vitamin B.

HERBS

Calendula, Comfrey, St John's Wort: These will promote healing and help to reduce scarring. Make an infusion to bathe the affected area or apply as an ointment.

HOMOEOPATHY

Arnica 200: One dose before and one dose after the operation to help with shock and promote rapid healing.
Gelsemium 30; One dose before operation for fear. Nervous and trembly feeling.
Phosphorus 30: For nausea and exhaustion following an anaesthetic. One or two doses.

AROMATHERAPHY
Calendula (Tagetes), Lavender, Patchouli, Sandalwood: Add a few drops of each oil to a wheatgerm oil base to promote healing and reduce scarring. Gently massage in on and around the affected area.

BACH FLOWER REMEDIES®

Rescue Remedy®: Take whenever necessary before and after; for anticipation, shock and trauma.

P

False Unicorn
(Chamaelirium Luteum)

PAIN

This is not an illness in itself, but a reaction to a physical or psychological cause, and it is that cause which one needs to identify and treat (getting rid of the sensation of pain without treating the cause can be beneficial in the short term, but it is often counter-productive in the long term).

An individual's response to pain varies from time to time as well as from person to person, and thus pains without a direct psychological cause should be referred to a holistic therapist. Those suffering from chronic pain also should seek advice. Obviously, acute pain should be treated according to its specific cause, but the following remedies may offer general help for pain-relief in the short term.

HERBS

Meadowsweet, St Johns Wort, Valerian, White Willow: All these have a mild pain relieving effect. Combine, infuse and drink a cupful every few hours.

HOMOEOPATHY

Arnica 6 or 30: Pain resulting from an injury or blow. Two or three doses.

Ferrum Phos 6X: Pain due to inflammation. Heat and redness may be present. One dose every few hours.

Hypericum 6 or 30: Pain following injury to parts rich in sentient nerves, e.g., fingers, toes, or to the spine. Two or three doses.

Kali Phos 6X: For pain involving nerve endings. Aggravated by nervousness and exhaustion. One dose every few hours.

Mag Phos 6X: Pains caused by muscular spasms and cramps. Tension. One dose every few hours.

AROMATHERAPY

Chamomile, Lavender, Marjoram: A few drops of these in a vegetable oil base and gently applied to the area will offer soothing relief. Alternatively, add a few drops to the bath.

BACH FLOWER REMEDIES®

Rescue Remedy®: Take internally as drops or apply externally onto the affected area.

Rescue Cream®: Apply to the affected area.

PILL (AFTER EFFECTS)

The advent of the contraceptive pill has enabled women to have greater sexual freedom, but at a loss. Although information on the side-effects of the pill has been available, it is often not taken seriously enough. Basically, the pill controls the hormonal system and, therefore, subtley controls the emotional side of the woman. The pill can be contributory in causing heart disease, thrombosis, cervical cancer, vaginal infections, weight gain and nausea.

When you stop taking the pill, the following remedies may assist in re-adjusting the hormonal balance of the body. If any problems persist, or you suspect you may be pregnant, consult a practitioner.

HERBS

Agnus Castus, Black Cohosh, Blue Cohosh, False Unicorn, Sarsaparilla: A mixture to assist in the functioning of the ovaries and re-balancing the hormones. Combine equal quantities, decoct and drink twice daily for four to five weeks. If you suspect you may be pregnant, do not take the herbs, but consult professional advice.

PALPITATIONS

Palpitations are caused either by the heart beating more forcibly, or the person's increased awareness of the heart beat. They are often transient and harmless and pass once the sufferer is able to relax. However, more prolonged episodes of palpitations, with rapid pulse, will need urgent medical assessment as this may indicate an underlying heart problem. Be cautious: if there is any departure from a previously stable pattern, seek medical advice, as an electrocardiogram can often provide a clear cut diagnosis.

The following remedies will offer relief in cases of mild palpitations where there is an obvious cause, such as nervous tension, and no other symptoms of heart trouble, e.g. chest tightness, dizziness, shortness of breath.

HERBS

Balm, Hawthorn, Lime Flowers, Motherwort, Passiflora: Combine the herbs and make an infusion using one heaped teaspoon of herbs to one cupful of boiling water, stand for ten minutes before straining. This may be drunk three times a day.

HOMOEOPATHY

Crataegus Tincture: A heart and circulation tonic. Take five drops in a wine glass of water three times a day.

124

Kali Phos 6X: Nervous palpitations. One dose every few hours as required.

AROMATHERAPY

Melissa, Neroli, Ylang Ylang: Add one or two drops of either of the oils to a warm bath, or add a few drops of each to a little vegetable oil base to use as a massage oil.

PLEURISY

Inflammation of the pleural membranes which surround the lungs. Pleurisy is often a secondary complaint associated with other lung diseases. The symptoms are pain on coughing, and when drawing in air. It may be accompanied with a fever.

Professional medical advice is essential when dealing with this complaint.

(See also: BRONCHITIS, CONVALESCENCE.)

PNEUMONIA

Inflammation of the lungs. This can occur on its own or as a secondary complaint of other illnesses.

Any sudden or long-term fever associated with a cough, especially with blood-tinged sputum, should arouse the suspicion of possible pneumonia. Immediate medical advice must be sought.

(See also: BRONCHITIS, CONVALESCENCE.)

125

POST-NATAL DEPRESSION

Most women will feel exhausted immediately after giving birth, and with successive disturbed nights, and the hormonal changes occurring at this time, re-adjustment to the new life with a baby can be worrying. Some women will experience actual depression after giving birth. If this becomes severe, or continues for more than a day or two, seek immediate professional advice. The following remedies will supplement professional help and relieve mild feelings of depression or post-natal blues.

(See also: CONVALESCENCE.)

HERBS

Agnus Castus, Balm, Lady's Slipper, Squaw Vine, Vervain, Wild Oat: A useful tonic to balance the hormones and nervous system. Take as tinctures or make a decoction and drink each morning and evening.

HOMOEOPATHY

Seek constitutional treatment according to individual symptoms.

AROMATHERAPY

Basil, Clary Sage, Geranium, Jasmine, Melissa: Combine two or three of the oils, or use separately, adding either a few drops to a bath, or in a massage base oil, and use regularly.

BACH FLOWER REMEDIES®

Study the Bach Flower literature (see Appendix) or consult an experienced practitioner to find the appropriate remedy. *Cherry Plum, Mustard, Olive, Willow* may be worth special consideration.

PREGNANCY

Whilst pregnancy is, of course, a completely natural process, it can place a lot of demands upon the emotions and body of a woman. Generally speaking, if you are feeling well, then it is better not to interfere in any way with the natural processes occuring at this time; but having said that, there is growing pressure on women today to keep active, and also have an entirely healthy and natural pregnancy and labour, which can feel quite overwhelming. Alternative medicine has many useful and safe treatments to assist a woman during this time, and the suggestions that follow will offer aid for certain problems; but ideally, a pregnant woman would benefit most from constitutional and specific treatment that could be offered by a qualified natural therapist.

There are several good organisations and much useful literature dealing with pregnancy these days. Consult the Appendix for a list of useful sources.

Of course, where possible, any drug medication should be avoided, as should stimulants, alcohol and cigarettes. There are many herbs and essential oils that, whilst perfectly safe to use at other times, may have an abortifacient effect and should be avoided during pregnancy. The following list comprises of those common herbs and oils which should not be used during pregnancy.

(See also: ANAEMIA, BREAST-FEEDING, CONSTIPATION, HEARTBURN, INDIGESTION, INSOMNIA, LABOUR, MORNING SICKNESS, POST-NATAL DEPRESSION, STRETCH MARKS, VARICOSE VEINS.)

HERBS TO AVOID DURING PREGNANCY

Aloes, Barberry, Black Cohosh, Bloodroot, Blue Cohosh, Buckthorn, Cascara Sagrada, Cinchona, Cottonroot, Greater Celandine, Juniper Liferoot, Male Fern, Mandrake, Pennyroyal, Pokeroot, Rhubarb, Rue, Saffron, Sage, Tansy, Thuja, Wormwood.

Generally speaking, this list includes those herbs acting as abortifacients, emmenagogues and strong laxatives. Really, any herb taken in therapeutic dosage should be specifically checked for use during pregnancy.

ESSENTIAL OILS TO AVOID DURING PREGNANCY

Basil, Camphor, Caraway, Cedar, Chamomile, Cinnamon, Fennel, Hyssop, Juniper, Nutmeg, Oreganum, Peppermint, Pennyroyal, Rosemary, Sage, Savoury, Thuja, Thyme, Wintergreen.

HERBS

Preparation for labour

Raspberry leaf: This tea drunk on a regular basis throughout the last three months of pregnancy will strengthen the uterine and pelvic muscles and help to make the birth easier. One heaped teaspoon to a cup of boiling water and infuse for ten minutes. Drink two or three times a day.

Squaw Vine: Drink regularly during the last two months of pregnancy to prepare the uterus for birth. One teaspoonful per cup of boiling water, drink a cupful daily. May be combined with *Raspberry leaves.*

After-birth bath

Comfrey, Marigold, St Johns Wort, Shepherd's Purse: Combine the above herbs and make into an infusion using one tablespoon to a pint of boiling water. After ten minutes strain, and pour the infusion into a bath of warm water and sit in the bath water for a soothing and healing bath. Alternatively, use the infusion, when cool, externally by applying to the perineum with cotton wool.

Healing

Calendula, Hypericum Tincture (Hypercal): Add a few drops of the tinctures to a small bowl of warm water. Apply with cotton wool to heal tears or stitches.

HOMOEOPATHY

Calc Fluor 6X: Gives elasticity to tissues, so helps prevent stretch marks and tones up the pelvic area. Also useful for the formation of healthy teeth and bones in the foetus. Take one dose twice a day for ten days at any time during pregnancy.

Ferrum Phos 6X: An alternative to synthetic iron tablets.

Encourages the body to assimilate iron more effectively. One dose two times a day for up to one month.

AROMATHERAPY

Rose, Marigold (Tagetes): A few drops of these oils in a vegetable base oil may be used for a pleasant, soothing massage at any time during pregnancy.

Wheatgerm Oil: This oil is rich in vitamin E and will help prevent stretch marks. It is a heavy oil and thus will be easier to use if combined with a lighter oil such as almond or apricot kernal oil. Massage into the skin regularly.

GENERAL SUPPLEMENTS

It can be necessary to increase the intake of iron during pregnancy. Rather than taking synthetic iron tablets which may cause indigestion or constipation, we suggest either: *Nettle Tea*; *Ferrum Phos* (see Homoeopathy); or *Floradix* — a herbally based iron-rich tonic available from health food shops.

PRE-MENSTRUAL TENSION

Hormonal changes are occurring all the time in women of menstruating age, and the individual's response will vary according to the constitution and general well-being of the body and emotions.

Increasing acceptance in our society of Pre-Menstrual Tension (PMT) may allow women to express and justify otherwise unacceptable emotions that are accentuated during these cyclic changes. Women that suffer distressing emotional symptoms prior to their periods could take this as an opportunity not to suppress these feelings, but to look at their general well-being in our stress-filled society; maybe with the help of a professional therapist.

Whilst we recognise that there is an inter-relationship between emotional and physical symptoms which should be explored for any condition, the following suggestions will help with the most commonly experienced physical symptoms that occur pre-menstrually; mainly due to salt and water accumulating in the tissues as a response to the hormonal secretions preceding menstruation. Physical symptoms frequently experienced by many women pre-menstrually include: nausea, headaches, bloatedness, swollen breasts, spots and other skin changes (see the relevant headings in the book).

(See also: MENSTRUAL PROBLEMS.)

HERBS

Agnus Castus, False Unicorn: These herbs have the effect of stabilising the hormones. Combine and make a decoction to drink three times a day as a course of treatment for up to three months. Alternatively take as tinctures.

Motherwort, Passiflora, Scullcap: Drink a combination of these herbs as an infusion three times a day when there are symptoms of anxiety and stress present.

Cramp Bark: This may be taken if there are cramping pains pressent.

Dandelion Leaves, Parsley: A combination of these infused and drunk three times a day can be used as a diuretic to ease bloatedness and other symptoms of water retention.

HOMOEOPATHY

There are homoeopathic remedies to help deal with these distressing symptoms, but one must consult a homoeopath for individual treatment to obtain full benefit.

AROMATHERAPY

Clary Sage, Geranium, Neroli, Rose: Any of these oils used as a few drops in the bath or in a massage oil will bring pleasant relief to distressing symptoms.

Juniper: A few drops diluted in vegetable oil and massaged in, or as a few drops in a bath, will have a diuretic effect.

130

BACH FLOWER REMEDIES®

These will undoubtedly be of assistance by working on the emotional causes of PMT. We suggest you refer to the appropriate literature, and choose the remedies most suitable for your needs.

GENERAL

Evening Primrose Oil: Either in capsule form, or taken as the oil itself, has proved to be of great benefit to many sufferers of the symptoms of PMT. As a guide to dosage, we suggest 1 × 500 mg per day for the first month, and then 1 × 500 mg per day for the appropriate ten days preceeding menstruation for succeeding months.
Similarly, many people have obtained benefit from vitamin therapy, in particular B6.

PSORIASIS

Over-production of skin cells usually presenting itself on bony areas of the body, e.g. shins, elbows or scalp. Symptoms include flaking of the skin, often accompanied by itching.

There is a hereditary factor to this disease, although it will also be aggravated by stress or trauma. Symptoms are often alleviated by sunshine and sea bathing. *Evening Primrose Oil* may also be of benefit. Take 1 × 500 mg capsule a day for two to three months.

Constitutional treatment is definitely recommended to get to the root of this disease.

HERBS

A qualified herbalist should be consulted for effective treatment, but the following herbs may assist.
Burdock Root, Red Clover, Sarsaparilla, Yarrow: A combination of

131

these herbs infused and taken three times daily over a period of time, up to three months.

AROMATHERAPY

HOMOEOPATHY

Consult a qualified practitioner.

AROMATHERAPY

Bergamot, Lavender, Sandalwood: Combine these oils; put a few drops in a bath or add to a vegetable oil base and massage into affected areas daily.

R

Poison Ivy
(Rhus Toxicodendron)

RHEUMATISM

Inflammation of the connective tissues covering the muscles, and of the tendons, also known as Myalgia, Fibrositis and Lumbago. The muscles in the area of the inflammation tighten as a defensive reaction and when this happens the nearby joint may become deformed. Hence, rheumatism and arthritis may often become confused.

Rheumatic fever is an acute form of rheumatism found mostly in children, heralded by sore throat and followed one to three weeks later by fever with transient joint pains, and occasionally muscular spasms. It should be treated by a qualified practitioner, due to the risk of inflammatory damage to the heart.

The treatment of rheumatism is similar to that of arthritis, and both are the result of an inappropriate diet which reduces the body's ability to eliminate toxic waste matter, combined with stress and tension in the lifestyle having its counterpart in the body, and a hereditary factor. Whilst the following suggestions will offer some alleviation from the discomfort of rheumatism, a holistic approach involving advice on diet, exercise and lifestyle is necessary to cure the problem. Constitutional treatment by a qualified holistic practitioner is recommended.

(See also: ARTHRITIS.)

133

HERBS

Internal

Bogbean: If the condition is aggravated in damp weather, add this to the following mixture.

Celery Seed, Dandelion, Meadowsweet, White Willow, Yarrow: A combination of these herbs will encourage the body to eliminate toxins and help with pain and inflammation.

Devil's Claw: This is a popular remedy for rheumatism. Soak a couple of pieces of the root in two cupfuls of water. The following morning boil up the root and water for ten to fifteen minutes, and then drink the liquid. Repeat daily.

External

Comfrey Oil, St Johns Wort Oil: Massage either of these oils over the affected area.

Rhus Tox Ointment: Rub into affected area.

HOMOEOPATHY

Arnica 6: Limbs ache as if beaten, affected parts feel sore and bruised. Rheumatic pains brought on by injury or over-exertion. One dose two times daily for up to ten days.

Bryonia 6: Heaviness of the limbs with redness and swelling of the joints. Patient feels compelled to keep the affected part still. Irritability. One dose twice daily for up to ten days.

Ferrum Phos 6X: Acute attacks of rheumatism. For pain, inflammation and congestion. One dose three times daily for up to ten days.

Nat Phos 6X: The acid neutralising tissue salt. Breaks up the harmful acids. One dose three times daily for up to ten days. May be taken in conjunction with *Nat Sulph*.

Nat Sulph 6X: Encourages removal of toxic charged fluids from the system. One dose three times daily for up to ten days.

Rhus Tox 6: Swelling and stiffness of limbs brought on by over-lifting or over-stretching. Also worse in cold, damp weather. Better from gentle motion, stiffens up during rest. One dose three times daily for up to ten days.

Juniper, Pine: A few drops of either of these oils in a bowl of warm water and use as a local bath or compress.

Benzoin, Eucalyptus, Lavender, Marjoram, Rosemary: Add a few drops of each oil to a vegetable base oil and massage into the area.

RINGWORM

A fungal infection of the skin which occurs on various parts of the body. The infection tends to spread outwards in a disc, the centre heals while the circumference is still active and forms a reddish circle. Scrupulous hygiene will be necessary to eliminate this problem as well as local healing applications. If the condition persists, constitutional treatment by a qualified therapist will be necessary.

HERBS

Echinacea, Marigold, Myrrh, Thuja: Combine tinctures of the above and apply locally to the area.

AROMATHERAPY

Lavender, Myrrh, Tea Tree: Apply any of the above, undiluted, to the affected area.

S

Orange Blossom
(Neroli)

SCABIES

A skin disease caused by a tiny parasitic insect which burrows under the skin, normally in the soft fleshy parts of the body, and never above the neck line. Scrupulous hygiene is imperative to prevent spreading. Before using orthodox treatment, some of the following could be tried:

HERBS

Poke Root, Tansy: A strong decoction should be made using 25 g of each herb to a pint and applied to the whole body twice a day.

HOMOEOPATHY

Staphisagria 6X: One dose three times a day for ten days in conjunction with external applications. Crawling sensation on the skin.

Sulphur 6: To improve quality of skin and help with itching, one dose morning and night for ten days.

AROMATHERAPY

Bergamot, Lavender, Peppermint, Rosemary, Tea Tree: Combine a few drops of each in a vegetable oil base and apply over the whole body.

136

SCIATICA

Pain in the area of the sciatic nerve i.e. back of the knee, calf or even extending to the back of the foot. The commonest cause is pressure on the spinal nerve which causes referred pain travelling down the sciatic nerve. Sometimes due to a slipped disc or to tension causing a trapped nerve aggravated by bad posture, stimulants, alcohol and tension. Acupuncture has been known to have good results for sciatica. Alexander Technique may be beneficial to correct posture if this is the root of the problem. Any manipulative therapy may help, e.g., Osteopathy, Chiropractice etc.

Prolonged episodes may result in damage to the sciatic nerve so careful treatment by an experienced practitioner is vital.

(See also: NEURALGIA.)

SHINGLES (HERPES ZOSTER)

Shingles is caused by a virus, similar to that which causes chicken pox. The distinguishing symptom is of painful clusters of blisters at the nerve endings. The patient feels generally unwell, and may be feverish during the acute attack. The pain may persist even when the blisters have gone.

An attack of shingles is often an indication of general debility and patients should have an improved diet and plenty of rest. Extra vitamins, and especially eating more foods rich in B vitamins will help.

The advice that follows applies to shingles on the chest, buttocks, etc.; shingles on the forehead or anywhere near the eyes should be treated only under the supervision of a medical practitioner.

137

HERBS

Internal

Lady's Slipper, Oats, Scullcap, St John's Wort, Vervain: Combine these nervine relaxants and tonics and make an infusion using a heaped teaspoon of dried herbs to a cupful of boiling water. Stand for ten minutes, strain, and drink a cupful three times a day.

External

Marigold, Plantain, St John's Wort: Make an infusion of these herbs using a tablespoon of herbs to a pint of boiling water. When cool, strain and apply to the affected areas using cotton wool. The tinctures may be diluted and used instead of an infusion.

HOMOEOPATHY

Ars Alb 6 or 30: Intense burning, with relief from warmth. Anxious and restless patient. One 30th potency a day for three days or one 6th potency three times a day for up to ten days.

Kali Phos 6X: Lightning pains along the nerves. A nerve nutrient useful to take after the initial attack. One dose three times a day for ten days.

Mezereum 6 or 30: Intolerable itching and painful eruptions aggravated by warmth and when in bed. Pain remains after the eruptions have gone. One 30th potency a day for three days or one 6th potency three times a day for up to ten days.

Rhus Tox 6 or 30: Intense itching with painful, watery blisters. Blisters on parts of the body covered with hair. One 30th potency a day for three days or one 6th potency three times a day for up to ten days.

AROMATHERAPY

Clary Sage, Eucalyptus, Geranium, Lavender, Peppermint: Choose one or more of the above and make a strong dilution in base oil to apply directly onto the affected areas. Alternatively, add five to ten drops of the chosen oil to a warm bath.

SHOCK

Technically shock is a reaction that occurs when the blood flow is reduced below the levels necessary to supply oxygen to the nervous system. Some degree of shock can occur after any injury, burn or illness that involves loss of blood or other body fluids. It can also occur during infection, allergic reaction or malfunction of the nervous system.

Symptoms of shock are: general weakness, cold, clammy, pale skin, a rapid, weak pulse, reduced alertness and shallow, irregular breathing. Nausea may also be present. Hot sweetened tea would help for minor shock.

One should suspect shock with any injury, and apply first-aid measures, whilst, if the injury appears severe, calling emergency aid. Reassure the patient, and get them to lay down with their feet slightly raised above the level of their head (except in the case of a head or chest injury where the head should be higher than the feet).

The following remedies will help for minor cases of shock, or may be administered whilst awaiting emergency medical treatment in more severe cases.

(See also: ACCIDENTS.)

HERBS

Balm, Chamomile, Peppermint, Scullcap: Make an infusion and sweeten with honey to drink when required.

HOMOEOPATHY

Aconite 30: Shock with extreme fear and panic. Nightmares following shock. Two or three doses.

Arnica 30 or 200: Shock from an accident or physical injury. Two or three doses.

Chamomilla 30: Shock where the patient is hysterical with the pain. Two or three doses.

139

China 30: Shock from loss of blood or other vital fluids. Two or three doses.

Ignatia 30: Shock from grief or fright with hysteria and fainting. Two or three doses.

AROMATHERAPY

Lavender, Melissa, Neroli, Peppermint: Use whichever is available. Hold under the patient's nose. Could also be used in a massage oil for delayed or emotional shock.

BACH FLOWER REMEDIES®

Rescue Remedy®: An invaluable aid at the time of shock. Take a few drops frequently, undiluted if necessary.

SINUSITIS

Infection or inflammation of the sinus cavities which often leads to increased mucous production. Symptoms include pain at the root of the nose, above or below the eyes, and a sensation of stuffiness in the head. Acute sinusitis may be accompanied by a fever and severe headache. It can become chronic and is often aggravated by colds, hayfever, emotional upset or damp weather. This should be treated constitutionally by a qualified practitioner. Acute attacks can often be managed by self-care, but any deterioration in the patient's condition is a signal for seeking medical advice.

We recommend a dairy-free diet to keep down mucous formation, and *Garlic* capsules to prevent infection.

HERBS

Echinacea, Elderflower, Eyebright, Golden Rod, Golden Seal, Marshmallow: Combine and infuse. This mixture drunk two times daily will help release blocked mucous and soothe inflammation.

140

HOMOEOPATHY

Bryonia 6 or 30: Heavy frontal headache; dryness and pressure sensation in nose; irritable. One dose of the 6 potency three times a day for five days or one dose of 30 a day for three days.

Kali Bich 6 or 30: Pressure or stuffed-up sensation at root of nose. Thick, stringy, yellow discharge. Localised frontal headache, especially over eyebrows; very painful. One 30 potency a day for three days, or one 6 three times a day for five days.

Kali Sulph 6 or 30: Nose bunged up; worse in warm room and evening; loss of taste; yellow catarrh. One 30 potency a day for three days or one 6 three times a day for five days.

Merc Sol 6 or 30: Infected catarrhal inflammation of frontal sinuses. Pain worse at night, purulent discharge, offensive taste in mouth. One 30 potency a day for three days or one 6 three times a day for five days.

Spigelia 6 or 30: Dryness of nose with post-nasal dripping. Neuralgic pains in cheeks or over eyes. One 30 potency a day for three days or one 6 three times a day for five days.

AROMATHERAPY

Eucalyptus, Pine, Thyme: Use a few drops of each of these oils as a steam inhalation.

SLEEPLESSNESS

(See: INSOMNIA.)

SORE THROAT

This is often the first indication of the onset of an illness. Most sore throats are self-limiting and symptoms will go with rest, fresh fruit and vegetables and plenty to drink. The following remedies will offer relief for any unacceptable discomfort. If symptoms persist or a high fever develops, call for professional advice.

(See also: COLDS, MUMPS, TONSILLITIS.)

HERBS

Red Sage: Make an infusion using a heaped teaspoon to a cup of boiling water, stand for ten minutes, strain and use as a gargle. This may also be drunk as a soothing tea.

Balm of Gilead, Echinacea, Poke Root: If the sore throat drags on, this mixture will be soothing and encourage the body to throw off the symptoms. Make a decoction simmering a teaspoon of herbs to a cupful of boiling water for ten minutes. Drink three times a day.

HOMOEOPATHY

Aconite 6 or 30; Sore throat preceding a cold or childhood illness. First stages. Two or three doses.

Belladonna 30: Sore throat and swollen, red tonsils. Fever with congested, red, hot face and skin. Take one dose of the 30th potency a day for three days.

Ferrum Phos 6X: Sore throat and hoarseness. Occurs when feeling run down. Redness and inflammation. One dose three times daily.

Hepar Sulph 30: Swelling of throat and glands in neck. Soreness. Sensation of fish bones in throat. Patient chilly and irritable. Take one dose of the 30th potency a day for three days.

Lachesis 30: Sensation of soreness and lump in the throat. Aggravated by swallowing. Pains move from left to right or are left-sided. Take one dose of the 30th potency a day for three days.

Merc Sol 30: Sore, raw throat, slow to improve. Feverishness worse at night. Swollen glands. Offensive breath. Painful

142

swallowing. Take one dose of the 30th potency a day for three days.

AROMATHERAPY

Lemon, Sage, Thyme: Dilute the oils in alcohol (vodka) and add a few drops to a cupful of warm water to use as a gargle or as a steam inhalation.

SPLINTERS

A foreign object beneath the skin. The object should be removed as quickly as possible to prevent infection.

HERBS

Hypercal Ointment: Put on a plaster to help draw out the splinter.
Marigold, St John's Wort: Either as tincture (known as *Hypercal*) or infusion. Soak the area concerned in the hot infusion or the tincture diluted in warm water.

HOMOEOPATHY

Hypericum 6 or 30: If it is very painful. Take three doses of the 6th potency a day for five days, or one dose of the 30th potency a day for three days.
Silica 6X: To encourage the body to expel the splinter. One three times a day for two to three days.

AROMATHERAPY

Lavender, Lemon: Apply neat over area to be treated and then put on a plaster to draw the splinter out.

143

SPRAINS AND STRAINS

An injury that tears or stretches supporting tissue of a joint; usually of ankles, wrists, fists or knees. To take strain off the affected joint whilst it heals, a supporting bandage may be required.

Cold water compressess may offer immediate relief. If symptoms appear at all severe, be aware that it may be a fracture and seek medical help.

(See also: ACCIDENTS, INJURIES.)

HERBS

Arnica, Comfrey, Witchazel: Use as tinctures or make an infusion for an external application — soak a cloth in the liquid and apply to the area as a compress.

Ointments

Arnica: Immediately after the injury for bruising and pain. Do not use on broken skin.

Rhus Tox: Injury to muscles. Swelling, pain and stiffness.

Ruta: Injury to ligaments and tendons. Massage well into the joint to promote rapid healing.

HOMOEOPATHY

Arnica 30: Use immediately after the injury for shock and to promote healing. Two or three doses.

Bellis Perennis 6: Muscles and joints sore and bruised. Swelling after an injury. After gardening. Three times a day for five days.

Hypericum 30: Violent pains in joint after injury. Nerve pains. Two or three doses.

Rhus Tox 6: Sprains that are sore, stiff and swollen. Area becomes stiff during rest and ameliorated by continued gentle movement. Painful on first moving. Three times a day for five days.

Ruta 6: Injury to ligaments, tendons and cartilage. Painful joints. Three times a day for five days.

144

AROMATHERAPY

Eucalyptus, Lavender, Rosemary: Combine oils and use on a warm cloth as a compress, or add the oils to a bowl of warm water and bathe the affected part.

STRETCH MARKS

Marks in the skin that form on fleshy parts such as thighs, buttocks, breasts and abdomen. They are formed when the skin has to accommodate weight loss or gain. Frequently occurring during pregnancy. There is an hereditary factor involved.

HOMOEOPATHY

Calc Fluor 6X: Gives elasticity to the skin. One morning and night for ten days. This may be taken during pregnancy.

AROMATHERAPY

Frankincense (Olibanum), Lavender, Lemongrass: Combined in a *Wheatgerm Oil* base (as it contains vitamin E), and massaged daily onto affected areas, or during pregnancy to areas most likely to be affected.

STYES

An infected boil or pimple on the eyelid without involvement of the eyeball and without any change in the vision of the eye. Inflammation erupts on the lid as a tender, red swelling. After a few days the stye usually comes to a head and discharges pus. Although sometimes painful, these are rarely dangerous, and

145

can heal by themselves. Recurring styes can be an indication of general debility, and toxicity, and unexpressed anger (emotion).

HERBS

Chamomile, Eyebright, Marigold: Combine, infuse and apply locally, as frequently as possible, or use diluted tinctures.

Burdock, Eyebright, Red Clover: Combine, infuse and drink three times daily for ten days. This will help to de-toxify the system and soothe the eyes.

HOMOEOPATHY

Apis 6 or 30: Painful styes with burning and stinging. Eyelid becomes red and swollen; worse from heat. One dose of 30 potency a day for two days or one 6 three times a day for five days.

Hepar Sulph 6 or 30: Stye hypersensitive to touch and cold air; splinter sensation in the eyelid, pain relieved by warm applications. Dosage as for *Apis.*

Pulsatilla 6 or 30: Unsightly inflammation, but not particularly painful. Discharge of bland yellow or green pus. Itching. Dosage as for *Apis.*

Silica 6X: Morning and night for ten days. Styes that never come to a head, or leave a hard lump in the eyelid.

Staphisagria 30: Styes come out in groups or are recurrent. Irritable. Eye feels dry. Two or three doses.

AROMATHERAPY

Chamomile: Soak cotton wool in a few drops mixed with warm water and hold over infected area.

SUNBURN

Exposure to the sun causes dehydration of the skin. To prevent painful burning and blistering, keep the skin protected with

146

sunscreening lotions and only expose yourself to the sun for short periods of time until accustomed to it. In the event of burning treat as for burns. There are a variety of well tried and effective skin treatments: bathing in cool *Chamomile* water; applying a mixture of *Calendula* Tincture and *Olive Oil*; *Lavender* essential oil applied undiluted; *Aloe Vera* gel applied directly; *St John's Wort* Oil or Ointment applied directly; *Urtica* Tincture or Ointment applied directly.

If the person becomes severely overheated, the cooling mechanism of the skin fails and it becomes hot and dry. The body temperature can rise dangerously. The person may feel dizzy, nauseated, weak, feverish and have a severe headache. Treat for shock, seek emergency care, and cool the person off as quickly as possible with cold water until temperature begins to drop. Avoid over-chilling and give a glass of cold water with half a teaspoon of salt to encourage perspiration, and equalise balance of body fluids.

HERBS

Chickweed, Nettle, Peppermint: A cooling combination of herbs. Make an infusion to drink as a tea or bathe on an over-hot area.

HOMOEOPATHY

Belladonna 30 or 200: Burning, dry, flushed skin. Feels feverish. Dilated pupils, throbbing headache. Two or three doses.
Glonoin 30 or 200: Bursting, pounding headache after exposure to sun. Two or three doses.
Nat Mur 6X: Several doses to encourage body fluids to return to normal.

AROMATHERAPY

Bergamot, Lavender: Cooling and soothing oils to apply in a massage base or to add a few drops to a cool bath.

T

Ginger
(Zingiber officinale)

TEETHING

Teething can be a distressing time for parents and infants. Teething symptoms vary according to the individual consitution; common symptoms are flushed cheek, slightly raised temperature, peevishness, skin eruptions due to higher levels of acidity, gnashing of gums, and an increased tendency to earache. The following remedies may assist, but if symptoms persist constitutional treatment will be required. Teething symptoms may mask the beginning of another illness, so consult a practitioner if there is any doubt.

HERBS

Chamomile: Make a weak infusion using one teaspoon of herb per half a pint of water. May be sweetened with honey if required. Allow the child to drink a tablespoon of infusion every four hours.

Marshmallow Root: Obtain the sticks for the child to chew on.

HOMOEOPATHY

Chamomilla 6X: Obtain in granule form or crush the tablet. Sprinkle a few granules or the powder onto the gums or into the mouth. Fretful, peevish child, one cheek flushed,

148

sleepless, demands attention. Slight fever. Greenish stools. Take one dose every four hours while symptoms persist.

Ferrum Phos 6X: Crush the tablet and sprinkle the powder onto the gums. For redness and inflammation and slight feverishness. Take one dose every four hours while symptoms persist.

Calc Phos, Kali Phos, Mag Phos 6X: Crush the tablet and place powder in mouth twice daily for ten days. For general debility and to promote healthy growth of the teeth.

THRUSH (CANDIDA)

Thrush is a yeast infection most commonly occuring in the mouth and the vagina, and can also occur in any folds of the skin, on the nipples, or in the bowel. Symptoms present with small red pimples becoming white patches, with a white discharge, itching and soreness in the area. This may be a sign of general debility, and sensitivity to fungal infections, or may be sexually transmitted. An increasingly common occurrence of thrush is after a course of antibiotics. Thrush in the mouth is most commonly found in babies, especially where there is an acid imbalance. It may be passed between the mouth and the nipple of the nursing mother. If vaginal thrush is aggravated by sexual contact, or if thrush is being passed between partners, then the use of a condom is advisable until the condition has improved.

The use of yogurt in the diet, and used externally, may be of benefit. Garlic capsules or fresh garlic have an anti-microbial effect. If thrush is recurrent, constitutional treatment will be necessary.

HERBS

Golden Seal, Lavender, Marigold, Myrrh, Thyme: Combine and make an infusion using equal parts for a vaginal douche. One dessertspoon of mixture to half a pint water. Leave standing until cool. Soak a piece of cotton wool in the infusion and use to liberally bathe the area.

Lavender, Myrrh: Combine equal parts, infuse and use as a mouthwash. One teaspoon of each tincture in warm water may be used instead.

HOMOEOPATHY

Kali Mur 6X: White discharge, white coated tongue. Thrush in infants. Three times a day for ten days.

Nat Phos, Nat Sulph, Silica: Acidity. Use in combination with a douche to eliminate thrush symptoms.

AROMATHERAPY

Lavender, Tea Tree, Thyme: Use externally. Ten drops to a pint of water used as a douche.

TONSILLITIS

Inflammation of the tonsils usually with streptoccocci bacteria present. It is most commonly found in children. Symptoms include: difficulty and pain when swallowing, white or red deposits on the tonsils and fever.

For an acute attack, treat as for fever and sore throat. Frequently recurring tonsillitis will require constitutional treatment from a qualified practitioner.

(See also: FEVER, SORE THROAT.)

TOOTHACHE

We can only suggest a few first-aid measures to apply locally as it is necessary to be treated by your dentist who will treat the source of the pain.

Calc Fluor 6X: Improves enamel of teeth prone to rapid decay. This is particularly useful to take if you do not use a toothpast containing fluoride and are prone to tooth decay. We recommend a course of *Calc Fluor 6X,* one twice daily for ten days, once a year.

HERBS

Marshmallow, Sage, Thyme: Make a strong infusion (three teaspoons per cup) and use as a mouthwash to help soothe inflammation and counter infection.

Cloves: Chew a few of these to release the analgesic oil that they contain.

HOMOEOPATHY

Arnica 6 or 30: Toothache following injury to the teeth or gums. Bruised soreness following a visit to the dentist. Two or three doses. Useful after tooth extraction.

Ferrum Phos 6X: Toothache with inflammation and soreness of gum, bleeding after extraction or after a blow to the area. One dose every two or three hours.

Kali Phos 6X: Severe pain in decayed or filled teeth, nagging dull toothache. One dose every two or three hours.

Mag Phos 6X: Severe toothache with shooting pains. Tooth sensitive to touch or cold air. One dose every two hours.

Silica 6X: Toothache due to gum boils or abscess. One dose three times daily.

AROMATHERAPY

Clove: Apply undiluted on cotton wool and place on affected area.

Peppermint: Though less effective, can be used in the same way.

These essential oils are not to be used for babies or young children.

151

TRAVEL SICKNESS

A condition brought on by motion disturbing the balance mechanism within the inner ear, causing feelings of nausea and sometimes vomiting. There is also a psychological factor as nervous anticipation of travelling itself can cause similar reactions.

General advice is to have fresh air, frequent light digestable meals, and during travelling to lie or sit with the head slightly tilted backwards (as in a deck chair!).

HERBS

Ginger: Chew the root, take ground *Ginger* in capsules, drink Ginger beer, or take diluted *Ginger* Tincture before and during the journey.

Meadowsweet, Peppermint Tinctures: Combine and add ten drops to a cupful of water. Drink a cupful every few hours.

HOMOEOPATHY

Cocculus 6: Severe nausea and vertigo. One dose before travel and repeat as necessary.

Petroleum 6: Dizziness and nausea aggravated by fumes. One dose before travel and repeat as necessary.

Tabacum 30: Boat sickness, worse in warm, severe nausea, violent vomiting. One dose before travel, and repeat as necessary.

AROMATHERAPY

Aniseed, Fennel, Ginger, Melissa, Peppermint: Use the essential oil of your choice undiluted on cotton wool or a tissue and inhale frequently.

U

Geranium~(Pelargonium)

ULCERS (EXTERNAL)

A persistent breach in a body surface. Their cause relies largely on where they are, but the failure to heal is the common link.

Varicose ulcers, found where there is poor circulation, are notoriously difficult to heal. Foot and leg exercises will help to encourage blood flow to the area. Professional medical care to advise about dressings is necessary. The following applications may also be tried for these and other slow-to-heal external lesions.

(See also: MOUTH ULCERS, WOUNDS.)

HERBS

Golden Seal, Hawthorn, St John's Wort, Shepherd's Purse, Stone Root, Yarrow: Combine and make an infusion to drink three times a day. This will stimulate circulation and promote healing.

Comfrey Root, Marigold, Marshmallow: A strong decoction of the above combination applied daily on clean lint to the area will reduce inflammation and promote healing. Simmer one dessertspoon of the herbs in half a pint of water for fifteen minutes; use when cool.

153

Tinctures

Calendula (Hypercal), Hypericum: Dilute ten drops of *Hypercal* in a cupful of boiled water. Wash the affected part with cotton wool dipped in the solution. Repeat twice daily.

AROMATHERAPY

Eucalyptus, Frankincense (Olibanum), Lavender: Add a few drops of any of these oils to a small bowl of warm boiled water. Stir the water, dip in a piece of clean lint, and place over the affected area.

ULCERS (INTERNAL)

Peptic ulcers refers to ulcers in the digestive tract, usually either gastric ulcers (stomach) or duodenal ulcers. Part of the mucous membrane of the stomach or duodenum becomes eaten into by the digestive juices which are highly acidic.

Emotional stress can promote a secretion of acid and is a cause of peptic ulcers. Other contributory factors are faulty diet (rich in fats and refined . carbohydrates), smoking, stimulants, and alcohol.

The symptoms always include stomach pains, which may occur anywhere in the upper abdomen, but usually in the midline. The pain is generally ameliorated by vomiting and usually for a short time after eating. Heartburn and nausea are also common symptoms. Most peptic ulcers bleed at times and may cause anaemia. This condition may be extremely serious and complications include: sudden and severe bleeding, perforation of the stomach or duodenum and narrowing of the outlet of the stomach. Any persistent pain associated with the stomach should be referred to a medical practitioner for diagnosis as other diseases may show similar symptoms.

The following remedies will almost certainly bring relief to the painful symptoms, but unless one is prepared to change the lifestyle and particularly the level of stress and the diet, any remedies will only temporarily alleviate the symptoms without really getting to the cause of the problem. Professional advice may well be a necessary part of the healing process.

(See also: GASTRITIS.)

HERBS

Comfrey, Golden Seal, Liquorice, Marigold, Marshmallow Root, Meadowsweet: A combination of these herbs made into an infusion using a heaped teaspoon to a cupful of boiling water will promote healing, reduce acidity and relieve pain. Take three times a day for six weeks.

Slippery Elm: This is a highly nutritious food as well as providing a mucilaginous lining for the digestive tract. Regular use of this herb taken as a teaspoon stirred into a cupful of warm water will relieve pain and discomfort.

For nervine mixtures see ANXIETY.

HOMOEOPATHY

Constitutional treatment by an experienced practitioner can be of definite aid in the healing of peptic ulcers.

AROMATHERAPY

Chamomile, Frankincense (Olibanum), Geranium, Marigold (Tagetes), Marjoram: Choose one or more of the above oils and add a few drops to a vegetable oil base. Massage into the abdomen. May be used in conjunction with other medication. Ideally, visit an aromatherapist for a relaxing and therapeutic massage.

V

Witchazel
(Hamamelis Virginiana)

VAGINAL INFECTIONS

The symptoms of a vaginal infection are irritation and/or an abnormal discharge. It is important to establish what exactly is causing the symptoms before treatment is possible, so seek medical advice. If a simple infection is diagnosed, treat as for THRUSH.

Vaginal infections are more common amongst women on the pill or after menopause, because the secretions of hormones at this time do not offer the same protection.

(See also: HERPES, THRUSH.)

VARICOSE VEINS

Swollen and distended veins in the leg caused by a combination of poor venous circulation, extra abdominal pressure, e.g. constipation, water retention, obesity, pregnancy and a herditary tendency. Prolonged periods of standing and lack of exercise and smoking are contributory factors. General measures to improve the problem include increased exercise, and a diet which will reduce the tendency to constipation — a wholefood diet including plenty of fresh fruit and vegetables is recommended. Resting with legs raised will help, together with giving up smoking and drinking less tea.

Rutin will help to build up the walls of the veins; these can be taken as a supplement or as buckwheat which is the main source of *Rutin*.

(See also: HAEMORRHOIDS.)

HERBS

External

Marigold, Witchazel: Can be made into a compress and used daily, or as a lotion applied onto the affected area.

Internal

Dandelion, Ginger, Horsechestnut, Lime Blossom: These herbs aid circulation, inflammation and are diuretic. Combine, using half as much *Ginger* as the other herbs, make an infusion using one teaspoon per cup, or use as tinctures diluted in water. Drink three cups a day for up to four weeks. If no improvement is seen, consult a practitioner.

HOMOEOPATHY

Calc Fluor 6X: To improve elasticity to the vein walls. Take one morning and night for ten days.
Hamamelis 6: Swollen, inflamed, painful, varicose veins, sore or prickling sensation in veins. Three times a day for a week.

AROMATHERAPY

Chamomile, Cypress, Lemon: Combine, add a few drops to a light vegetable base oil and massage into legs around, rather than on, the veins, or use in the bath.

157

VOMITING

A reflex action with reversal of the normal movements of the muscles in the wall of the stomach. The reflex is clearly protective when it is set off by an irritant in the stomach or by overloading.

Repeated, forcible or sustained vomiting is always a serious symptom. It may indicate an emergency such as obstruction of the abdomen or poisoning, and it may lead to dehydration. Call emergency medical aid, whilst making sure the person is lying on their side so they cannot inhale the vomit, if they are unable to remain upright. Speed of action is essential with infants as they dehydrate so quickly.

For mild vomiting with an obvious cause, we suggest the following.

(See also: HANGOVERS, MORNING SICKNESS, NAUSEA, TRAVEL SICKNESS.)

HERBS

Balm, Chamomile, Meadowsweet: Make an infusion of the above and sip the tea to reduce nausea and soothe the stomach.

HOMOEOPATHY

Aethusa 6 or 30: Infant vomits their usual milk. Milk comes up in curds. If severe get immediate medical advice. Two or three doses.

Ars Alb 6 or 30: Vomiting and purging. Sips hot or cold drinks. Fearful and restless. Two or three doses.

Bryonia 6 or 30; Vomiting of solid food immediately after eating. Nausea and vomiting much better when lying absolutely still. Thirsty. Two or three doses as required.

Ipecac 6 or 30: Vomiting with constant nausea, not relieved by the vomiting. Clean tongue. Two or three doses as required.

Nux Vomica 6 or 30: Patient feels better for a while immediately after vomiting, then nausea builds up again; worse after overloading the stomach; chilly and irritable. Two or three doses as required.

Pulsatilla 6 or 30: Stomach feels heavy. Aggravated by rich, fatty food. Thirstless. Feels sorry for themselves. Two or three doses.

Phosphorus 6 or 30: Great thirst for cold water that is vomited as soon as it reaches the stomach. Restless and anxious. Better for resting, burning in stomach. Two or three doses.

AROMATHERAPY

Basil, Peppermint, Melissa: Add a few drops of the oil in a vegetable base and massage into the abdomen.

W

Bearberry ~ (Arctostaphylos uva-ursi)

WARTS AND VERRUCAE

A wart is a growth on the skin that may be either hard or soft and fleshy. Warts are found in association with a virus which enters the body through a break in the skin, however, only a susceptible person will actually grow a wart which presents the probable need for constitutional treatment to properly eliminate the tendency to grow warts.

The most common sites for warts are fingers, knees, face and genitals.

Plantar warts (verrucae) are found on the soles of the feet and may become painful. They usually have a visible dark core. Treatment will be necessary to prevent them spreading.

The following remedies have been found to be successful where the warts are of a superficial nature. If they do not disappear, then the need for constitutional treatment to treat the tendency to produce warts is apparent.

HERBS

Dandelion: Squeeze the milky white sap from a stalk of fresh *Dandelion* onto the wart every day.

Garlic: Rub the wart with a slice from a peeled clove of *Garlic* every evening.

160

Tinctures

Thuja: Dab on three times a day.

AROMATHERAPY

Lemon, Tea Tree: Dab on either of these oils, neat, twice daily.

WATER RETENTION

Water retention is caused by the accumulation of fluid in the tissues. There are several distinct causes of water retention. In heart failure the water will accumulate in the legs, and in the cavity of the abdomen (ascites). Liver disease will cause water retention in the cavity of the abdomen. Salt retention will cause the tissues to retain more water; this is the cause of water retention associated with pregnancy or pre-menstrual tension where the change in hormone levels causes the body to retain more salt. Starvation and kidney disease will also cause water retention.

It becomes obvious that water retention is only curable by treating the cause and it is important to establish what the cause is. Salt will aggravate any water retention, therefore, a salt-free diet is advisable. The following remedies comprise of some well-tried diuretics that may be used in consultation with your practitioner.

(See also: CELLULITE, CIRCULATION, JET LAG.)

HERBS

Cornsilk, Dandelion, Uva Ursi, Yarrow: Combine two or three of the above and make an infusion using a teaspoon of the herbs to a cup of boiling water. Drink three times daily. The most useful is probably *Dandelion* because it is naturally rich in potassium, and all diuretics tend to cause a loss of potassium from the body.

HOMOEOPATHY

Constitutional treatment must be sought.

AROMATHERAPY

Cypress, Juniper, Rosemary: Dilute a few drops of each in a massage base oil, or add a couple of drops of one of them into the bath. These oils are not to be used during pregnancy.

WHOOPING COUGH

This is an infectious disease which affects the mucous membranes of the air passages, and usually occurs in children. The incubation period is around one week, and the initial symptoms are a sore throat and a cold.

After a week a violent, convulsive cough, which may be accompanied by vomiting, will occur. This can be very distressing, as during a coughing bout the child may not have time to draw in air and the 'whoop', so characteristic of the disease, is heard as the child struggles to inhale. This may not happen during a mild attack, but careful treatment and professional help should always be sought for whooping cough as damage can occur to the lungs or pneumonia may set in, especially in babies.

The following remedies must be used as an adjunct to medical supervision, and not replace it.

HERBS

Aniseed, Coltsfoot, Elecampane, Horehound, Linseed, Liquorice, Thyme: Combine the above and make an infusion using two teaspoons of herbs to a cup of boiling water. Leave to stand for ten minutes, then strain and add honey to taste.

Dosage

Babies: One teaspoon of infusion every four hours.
6 months to 5 years: Two teaspoons every four hours.
Children over 5 years: One tablespoon every four hours.

HOMOEOPATHY

Bryonia 6 or 30: Cough after eating and drinking. Child vomits. Dry, hard, painful cough, dreads the pain of the cough. One dose of 30th potency a day for three days, or three doses of 6th potency a day for five days.

Carbo Veg 6 or 30: Attacks of tormenting, choking cough. Face is blushed. Expectoration thick, yellow and profuse. Child craves fresh air. One dose of 30th potency a day for three days, or three doses of 6th potency a day for five days.

Coccus Cacti 6 or 30: Regular paroxysms of violent, tickling, racking cough ending in vomiting or raising of much clear, ropy mucous. Mucous hangs from the mouth. Purple face. Worse lying down. One dose of 30th potency a day for three days, or three doses of 6th potency a day for five days.

Drosera 6 or 30: Spasmodic, prolonged and incessant cough, followed by retching and vomiting. One dose of 30th potency a day for three days, or three doses of 6th potency a day for five days.

Ipecac 6 or 30: Cough violent and incessant. With every breath the child stiffens out, becomes blue or red in the face, and finally vomits. One dose of 30th potency a day for three days, or three doses of 6th potency a day for five days.

Pertussin 30: This is considered by some to be a homoeopathic prophylactic against whooping cough. Give the child one dose a week during a whooping cough outbreak, or consult your practitioner.

Veratrum Alb 6 or 30: Continuous violent, barking cough. Child desires ice and sour foods. One dose of 30th potency a day for three days, or three doses of 6th potency a day for five days.

Finding the right homoeopathic remedy for whooping cough is not easy, and seeking professional guidance will bring the best results.

163

Basil, Cypress, Thyme: Place a few drops on a piece of cotton wool and put on the pillow near the child, or burn on an essential oil burner in the room. One drop of each may be added to a little vaseline and rubbed onto the chest.

WIND

(See: COLIC, FLATULENCE.)

WORMS

The following treatment is recommended for threadworms and roundworms, tapeworms must be treated professionally. Parasitic worms are a fairly common complaint, mostly in children. It is estimated that about 30 per cent of English children suffer from intestinal worms, mostly threadworms. These are passed on through oral infection from the anus where the worms lay their eggs. The life cycle of the egg in threadworms is about ten days, and so treatment must be aimed at breaking this cycle as well as alleviating the symptoms.

The symptoms of intestinal worms are irritability, boring of the nose with the fingers, and most markedly an itchy anus, which will be worse in the evening when the worms come out to lay their eggs. Diagnosis may be confirmed by observing the worms in the stools or around the anus in the evening.

Treatment requires scrupulous hygiene, paying particular attention to underwear, sheets and bed linen. The child should wear closely fitting underwear at night so they cannot inadvertently scratch the anus; wash the hands with hot soapy water, and scrub the nails after every visit to the lavatory. It will also be helpful to eat foods that the worms do not like, such as raw carrots, apples, onions, garlic and pumpkin seeds. Worms live on sugars so all foods containing sugar or even natural sweeteners such as malt or honey should be avoided.

Calendula Ointment or vaseline should be applied to the anus every evening to prevent the worms from laying their eggs and to relieve the itching.

HERBS

Herbs which will kill worms are anthelmintics, these should be combined with a mild laxative to eliminate the worms.

Balmony, Liquorice, Quassia, Wormwood: A very bitter but effective tea. Make a decoction and drink three times a day for three weeks. An enema of the herbs can be successful, but this is only advisable for adults.

HOMOEOPATHY

Cina 200: Threadworms and roundworms. Twisting pains at the naval, itching at the anus, worse in the evenings. Irritable child, teeth grinding. One dose at bedtime, one the following morning; this may be repeated in ten days.

Nat Phos 6X: A course of this, one dose morning and night for ten days is a useful follow-up to either of the above remedies. It will help to rebalance the acid condition in the intestine, which becomes unbalanced with worms.

Tellurium 30: Itching is worse after passing stool. Pinching pains in abdomen. One dose a day for three days.

AROMATHERAPY

Eucalyptus, Lavender: Add a couple of drops to vaseline and apply around the anus.

WRINKLES

Age, insomnia, weight loss, excessive sun, smoking, a hard life and hereditary tendencies (skin type), will all be significant in the development of wrinkles (or character lines).

It is the general level of mental and physical health which is most important to deal with. In order to lessen the process of forming wrinkles the following applications will help to allay the effects of ageing, and keep the skin supple:

Wheatgerm Oil: This is rich in natural vitamin E which will help to keep the skin in good condition. Take two to four capsules a day, or apply the oil externally to the skin. (See also: AGEING.)

AROMATHERAPY

Carrot, Frankincense (Olibanum), Neroli, Rose, Sandalwood: Add a few drops of each to a light vegetable oil base and gently massage into the skin. A little wheatgerm oil, macademia nut oil or hazelnut oil may also be added.

Appendix

BACH FLOWER REMEDIES

The list below is intended only as an aid to memory and for general enlightenment — one must not prescribe from this list, otherwise disappointing results can ensue. See the Bibliography for essential books on the subject, especially *The Twelve Healers* which offers Dr Bach's original descriptions.

1 *Agrimony*   Those who hide worries behind a brave face.
2 *Aspen*   Apprehension for no known reason.
3 *Beech*   Critical and intolerant of others.
4 *Centaury*   Weak willed; exploited or imposed upon.
5 *Cerato*   Those who doubt their own judgement, seeks confirmation of others.
6 *Cherry Plum*   Uncontrolled, irrational thoughts.
7 *Chestnut Bud*   Refuses to learn by experience — continually repeats same mistakes.
8 *Chicory*   Over possessive — (self-centred) — clinging and over-protective especially of loved ones.
9 *Clematis*   Inattentive, dreamy, absent-minded.
10 *Crab Apple*   The 'Cleanser'. Self disgust/detestation. Ashamed of ailments.
11 *Elm*   Overwhelmed by inadequacy and responsibility.
12 *Gentian*   Despondency.
13 *Gorse*   Pessimism, defeatism — 'Oh what's the use!'.
14 *Heather*   Talkative (obsessed with own troubles and experiences).
15 *Holly*   Hatred, envy, jealousy, suspicion.
16 *Honeysuckle*   Living in the past — nostalgic. Home-sickness.
17 *Hornbeam*   'Monday morning' feeling — procrastination.
18 *Impatiens*   Impatience, irritability.
19 *Larch*   Lack of self-confidence. Feels inferior. Fears failure.
20 *Mimulus*   Fear of *known* things. Shyness, timidity.
21 *Mustard*   'Dark cloud' that descends, making one saddened and low for no known reason.

22 *Oak* Normally strong/courageous, but no longer able to struggle bravely against illness and/or adversity.

23 *Olive* Fatigued — drained of energy.

24 *Pine* Guilt complex — blames self even for mistakes of others. Always apologising.

25 *Red Chestnut* Obsessed by care and concern for others.

26 *Rock Rose* Suddenly alarmed, scared, panicky.

27 *Rock Water* Rigid minded, self denying.

28 *Scleranthus* Uncertainty/indecision/vacillation. Fluctuating moods.

29 *Star of Bethlehem* For all the effects of serious news, or fright following an accident, etc.

30 *Sweet Chestnut* Absolute dejection.

31 *Vervain* Over-enthusiasm — fanatical beliefs.

32 *Vine* Dominating / inflexible / tyrannical / autocratic / arrogant. Usually good leaders.

33 *Walnut* Assists in adjustment to transition or change, e.g. puberty, menopause, divorce, new surroundings.

34 *Water Violet* Proud, reserved, enjoys being alone.

35 *White Chestnut* Persistent unwanted thoughts. Pre-occupation with some worry or episode. Mental arguments.

36 *Wild Oat* Helps determine one's intended path in life.

37 *Wild Rose* Resignation, apathy.

38 *Willow* Resentment, embitterment, 'poor old me!'.

39 *RESCUE REMEDY* A combination of Cherry Plum, Clematis, Impatiens, Rock Rose, Star of Bethlehem. All purpose emergency composite for effects of anguish, examinations, going to the dentist, etc. Comforting, calming and reassuring to those distressed by startling experiences.

©BACH CENTRE, UK 1950/62/80/83/85/86/87
Printed with kind permission of the Bach Centre, UK.

SUPPLIERS

When purchasing items for medicinal purposes it is essential to use products of good quality.

Herbs, where possible, should be organically grown, and as fresh as possible. There are many well-established herbal retailers in Britain and America.

Homoeopathic remedies must be carefully prepared and stored.

Essential oils must be pure and of natural origin. Synthetic oils will not produce satisfactory therapeutic results, and may be damaging.

Check with your retailer that their oils are definitely unadulterated essential oils.

All the products mentioned in this book are available from branches of Neal's Yard Remedies. A mail order service is also available. For details telephone 081–379 0705.

Neal's Yard Remedies,
15 Neal's Yard,
Covent Garden,
London WC2.
Tel: 071–379 7222.

Neal's Yard Remedies,
Chelsea Farmers Market,
Sydney Street,
London SW3 6NR.
Tel: 071–351 6380.

Neal's Yard Remedies,
68 Chalk Farm Road,
London NW1 8AN.
Tel: 071–284 2039.

Neal's Yard Remedies,
2A Kensington Gardens,
Brighton BN1 4AL.
Tel: (0273) 601464.

Neal's Yard Remedies,
126 Whiteladies Road,
Clifton,
Bristol BS8 2RP.
Tel: (0272) 466034.

Neal's Yard Remedies,
26 Lower Goat Lane,
Norwich NR2 1EL.
Tel: (0603) 766681.

Neal's Yard Remedies,
5 Golden Cross Walk,
Cornmarket Street,
Oxford OX1 3EU.
Tel: (0865) 245436.

Neal's Yard Remedies,
Little Priory,
Fore Street,
Totnes,
Devon TQ9 5HJ.
Tel: (0803) 864640.

In the USA most products should be available in local health food stores. Where they are not, contact one of the organisations whose addresses are on the following pages to find out about reputable suppliers.

CONTACTS

HERBS

UK:

National Institute of Medical Herbalists,
41 Hatherly Road,
Winchester,
Hants.
Tel: (0962) 68776.

British Herbal Medicine Association,
Lane House,
Cowling,
Keighley,
W. Yorkshire DB22 0LX.

USA:

Dr Christopher Enterprises,
PO Box 352,
Provo, UT.84601.

East–West Herb Courses,
c/o Michael Tierra,
Box 712,
Santa Cruz,
CA.950061.

HOMOEOPATHY

UK:

British Homoeopathic Association,
27a Devonshire Street,
London W1N 1RJ.
Tel: 071–935 2163

Society of Homoeopaths,
11a Bampton Street,
Tiverton, Devon,
EX16 6HH.
Tel: (0884) 255117.

College of Homoeopathy,
26 Clarendon Rise,
London SE13.
Tel: 081–852 0573.

North America:

National Center for Homoeopathy,
1500 Massachusetts Avenue, NW,
Washington, DC 20005.

US Homoeopathic Association,
6560 Backlick Road,
Springfield, VA 22150.

International Foundation for Homoeopathy,
1141 NW Market Street,
Seattle, WA 98107.

Pan–American Homoeopathic Medical Congress,
Francisco del Paso y Troncoso Edifico 166,
Entrada D. Unidad Kennedy,
Mexico 9, D.F.

Boericke and Tafel, Inc. (Suppliers),
1011 Arch Street,
Philadelphia, PA 19107.

AROMATHERAPY

UK:

International Federation of Aromatherapists,
46 Dalkeith Road,
London SE21 8LS.

The Association of Tisserand Aromatherapists,
31 Craven Street,
London WC2.
Tel: 071–930 3340.

Guild of Aromatherapy Practitioners,
59 Murray Road,
London SW19.

London School of Aromatherapy,
PO 780,
London NW6 5EQ.

BACH FLOWER REMEDIES®

UK:

Dr Edward Bach Centre,
Mount Vernon,
Sotwell,
Wallingford,
Oxfordshire OX10 0PZ.
Tel: (0491) 39489.

USA:

Ellon (Bach USA) Inc.,
PO Box 320,
Woodmere,
NY 11598.
Tel: 516 593 2206.

Bibliography

Herbs

Gosling, N., *Successful Herbal Remedies*, Wellingborough, England: Thorsons, 1985.

Grieve, M., *A Modern Herbal*, London: Penguin, 1931.

Griggs, B., *The Home Herbal*, London: Pan, 1982.

Hoffman, D., *The Holistic Herbal*, Findhorn, Scotland: Findhorn Press, 1983.

Kloss, J., *Back to Eden*, California, USA: Back to Eden Books, 1949.

Mills, S.Y., *The Dictionary of Modern Herbalism*, Wellingborough, England: Thorsons, 1985.

Tierra, M., *The Way of Herbs*, Santa Cruz, USA: Orenda/United Press, 1980.

Homoeopathy

Clarke, J.H., *The Precriber*, Saffron Walden, England: Health Science Press, 1972.

Cummings, S., Ullman, D., *Everybody's Guide to Homeopathic Medicines*, Los Angeles, USA: Tarcher, 1984.

Lessel, C.B., *The Biochemic Handbook*, Wellingborough, England: Thorsons, 1984.

Panos, M., Heimlich, J., *Homeopathic Medicine at Home*, Los Angeles, USA: Tarcher, 1980.

Phatak, S.R., *Materia Medica of Homoeopathic Medicines*, Delhi, India: IBPS, 1977.

Shepherd, D., *Homoeopathy for the First Aider*, Saffron Walden, England: Health Science Press, 1945.

Speight, P., *Before Calling the Doctor*, Saffron Walden, England: Health Science Press, 1976.

Speight, P., *Homoeopathic Remedies for Children*, Saffron Walden, England: Health Science Press, 1983.

Vithoulkas, G., *Medicine of the New Man*, New York: Arco, 1979.

Aromatherapy

Arnould Taylor, W.E., *Aromatherapy for the Whole Person*, Cheltenham, England: Stanley Thornes, 1981.

Davis, P., *Aromatherapy: An A-Z*, Saffron Walden, England: C.W. Daniel, 1988.

Jackson, J., *Aromatherapy*, New York: Henry Holt, 1986.

Price, S., *Practical Aromatherapy*, Wellingborough, England: Thorsons, 1983.

Tisserand, R., *The Art of Aromatherapy*, Saffron Walden, England: C.W. Daniel, 1977.

Valnet, J., *The Practice of Aromatherapy*, Saffron Walden, England: C.W. Daniel, 1980.

Worwood, V.A., *Aromantics*, London: Pan, 1987.

Bach Flower Remedies

Bach, E., *Heal Thyself*, Saffron Walden, England: C.W. Daniel, 1931.

Bach, E., *Twelve Healers*, Saffron Walden, England: C.W. Daniel, 1933.

Barnard, J., *A Guide to the Bach Flower Remedies*, Saffron Walden, England: C.W. Daniel, 1979.

Chancellor, P.M., *Handbook of the Bach Flower Remedies*, Saffron Walden, England: C.W. Daniel, 1971.

Hyne Jones, T.W., *Dictionary of the Bach Flower Remedies*, Saffron Walden, England: C.W. Daniel, 1976.

Wheeler, F.J., *The Bach Remedies Repertory*, Saffron Walden, England: C.W. Daniel, 1952.

Index

ARKANA – NEW-AGE BOOKS FOR MIND, BODY AND SPIRIT

A selection of titles

With over 200 titles currently in print, Arkana is the leading name in quality new-age books for mind, body and spirit. Arkana encompasses the spirituality of both East and West, ancient and new, in fiction and non-fiction. A vast range of interests is covered, including Psychology and Transformation, Health, Science and Mysticism, Women's Spirituality and Astrology.

If you would like a catalogue of Arkana books, please write to:

Arkana Marketing Department
Penguin Books Ltd
27 Wright's Lane
London W8 5TZ